Third Edition

Patient Education

A Practical Approach

Kate Lorig
and Associates

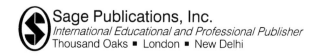

Sage Publications, Inc.
International Educational and Professional Publisher
Thousand Oaks ▪ London ▪ New Delhi

For information address:

Sage Publications, Inc.
2455 Teller Road
Thousand Oaks, California 91320
E-mail: order@sagepub.com

Sage Publications Ltd.
6 Bonhill Street
London EC2A 4PU
United Kingdom

Sage Publications India Pvt. Ltd.
M-32 Market
Greater Kailash I
New Delhi 110 048 India

Printed in the United States of America

Library of Congress Cataloging-in-Publication Data

Lorig, Kate.
    Patient education: A practical approach / by Kate Lorig and associates.– 3rd ed.
    p. cm.
    Includes bibliographical references and index.
    ISBN 0-7619-2290-3 (p: acid-free paper)
    1. Patient education. I. Title.
    R727.4 .L67 2000
    615.5'071–dc21   00-010036

01 02 03 04 05 06 10 9 8 7 6 5 4 3 2 1

Acquiring Editor:	Margaret H. Seawell
Editorial Assistant:	Heidi Van Middlesworth
Production Editor:	Nevair Kabakian
Editorial Assistant:	Candice Crosetti
Typesetter/Designer:	Rebecca Evans /Janelle LeMaster
Indexer:	Teri Greenberg
Cover Designer:	Michelle Lee

Contents

Preface

This book is designed to solve problems, give practical advice, and build new skills. It is for health professionals who are not skilled in patient education but need to know where to start and how to proceed. It may also be useful to students who are just beginning to learn the tricks of the trade. If you use it as a text, it will take you step by step through the process of conceptualizing, designing, implementing, and evaluating patient education programs. It will also help you with gaining accreditation for your organization from the Joint Commission on Accreditation of Healthcare Organizations (JCAHO).

Over the past several years, I have been asked to conduct many patient education skills-building workshops. Some of these have been sponsored by the Veterans Administration and the American Hospital Association in the United States, others by the Arthritis Societies of New Zealand and Canada, the Arthritis Foundations of various states in Australia, and the Department of Rehabilitation at the University of Göteborg in Sweden. Others have been sponsored by the Health Education Society in British Columbia and the Society for Public Health Education in Seattle, Washington. I have also been fortunate to consult with many fine colleagues in the Kaiser Permanente health care system.

During this same time, I have been running the Patient Education Research Center at Stanford University. This center has involved hundreds of community-based courses for thousands of people with arthritis and other chronic diseases, including heart disease, lung diseases, stroke, diabetes, back pain, and AIDS. Our research has shown that patient education can change behaviors, improve health status, and reduce health care costs.

This book is a result of all the above activities. It is a collection of the bits and pieces designed for my workshops and reflects my experiences and those of my colleagues here at Stanford and the real-life experiences of the workshop participants. By including a large section on health education theory, I hope to help practitioners use theory in everyday practice. In short, this is a "how-to" guide to patient education that has grown out of my work over the past decade. I have tried to make suggestions that will have immediate relevance to practice. At the same time, many of you will want more information. You can find such information by exploring the works listed in the brief bibliographies provided at the ends of the chapters in this volume.

Please visit our Web site at http://www.stanford.edu/group/ perc. We welcome your suggestions and comments.

Acknowledgments

Books don't just happen. This book is no exception. Over the years, many people have been very helpful. Milton Chernin was the first to suggest that I might write a book. I regret that I was too slow to allow him to see the finished product. Many people have helped me learn about patient education. These include Carol D'Onofrio, Wendy Cuneo, Larry Green, Rusty Rosenstock, Charles Watson, Judith Miller, Barbara Giloth, Sam Radelfinger, Helen Ross, Rosemary Pries, David Sobel, Michael Von Korff, David Sobel, Laurie Doyle, and Mary Hobbs. Over the years, Godfry Hochbaum gave more wisdom and support than he could ever know.

For the past 21 years, I have had five Stanford mentors and colleagues who have supported my work, tried to keep me on track, and at the same time allowed me to explore uncharted territory. My very special thanks to Halsted Holman, James Fries, Albert Bandura, Diana Laurent, and Virginia González.

Added to these professionals are the hundreds of people who have attended the patient education workshops I have conducted in the United States, Canada, Australia, New Zealand, Great Britain, South Africa, Singapore, and Sweden. You have asked important questions and have served as my guides for moving patient education from the ivory tower of academe to the clinical setting. In addition, you have given me many ideas based on your practice.

Finally, there is a group of friends and colleagues who have written, typed, proofread, edited, critiqued, and in many other ways made this book more readable. My deepest appreciation to Jean Goeppinger, Cecilia and Leonard Doak, Tom Prohaska, Lynn Gordon, Gloria Samuel, Margo Harris, Jenny Davidson, and Ian Fraser.

Introduction

Throughout this book, I talk about "patient" education. The reason I use the word *patient* is that this is not a book about health promotion or disease prevention, although much of what is discussed here could be applied to such programs. Rather, it is about *patients*–people who have defined health problems, such as high blood pressure, cancer, diabetes, or AIDS. Usually, when someone is receiving medical care for a condition, we call him or her a patient. This is especially true in hospitals and clinics. However, this same person with his or her illness is often found getting on with life in the community. In this case, he or she becomes a person with diabetes, high blood pressure, AIDS, or whatever. Somehow, saying "education for people with _____ " is rather awkward. Thus, for literary purposes and to save trees, I talk about patient education.

Patient education is any set of planned, educational activities designed to improve patients' health behaviors, health status, or both. Notice that there is nothing in this definition about improving knowledge. Activities aimed at improving knowledge are

xiii

patient teaching. Changes in knowledge may be necessary before we can change behaviors or health status. However, just
because someone has correct knowledge does not mean that
he or she will change. If all we needed were knowledge, there
would be no smokers, overweight people, or people eating high-
cholesterol foods. Patient education is much more than knowledge change. On the other hand, a person can have good health
behaviors without a lot of knowledge. Most of us brush our teeth
daily, but only a few of us can tell someone else quickly how
many teeth we have.

The purposes of patient education are to maintain and
improve health and, in some cases, to slow deterioration. These
purposes are met through changes in behaviors, mental attitudes, or both. Increased compliance with medication taking,
decreased pain, shorter hospital stays, and decreased depression
are all reasonable goals for patient education programs.

In recent years, patient education has become increasingly
complex because it is no longer considered enough for patients
to learn and practice specific skills. Rather, patients must manage
their own diseases. Such patient self-management differs from
previous approaches in that self-management education must
assist patients in gaining both skills and, more important, the
confidence to apply these skills on a day-to-day basis. It must
also help the patient to cope with changing roles and changing emotions. The three most distinctive features of the self-
management model for patient education are (a) dealing with
the consequences of disease—illness—not just the physiological
disease; (b) being concerned with problem solving, decision
making, and patient confidence, rather than with prescription
and adherence; and (c) placing patients and health professionals
in partnership relationships. Health professionals are primarily
responsible for the medical management of the disease, and the
patient is primarily responsible for the day-to-day management
of the illness. The key to full partnership is continual communication between patient and health professional.

Now that we have defined *patient* and *patient education,* there is one term left—*planned educational activities.* Patient education does not just happen; it is planned. This book is about the planning of patient education activities.

◘ HOW TO USE THIS BOOK

Being a patient educator is a little like being a jack-of-all-trades. Often, you are called upon to design something such as a program or a one-on-one intervention. Other times, you are asked to fix something—to answer questions such as "Why don't people come to my program?" and "Why don't the patients do what I tell them to do?" Still other times, you are asked to evaluate patient education. Another role for the patient educator involves referring patients and others to resources, answering questions such as "Where do I get information on Parkinson's disease?" and "Where can I get a slide projector?" Finally, you may be asked to help prepare your facility for accreditation. Sometimes you are expected to put all of these roles together and create, implement, and evaluate entire programs. This book is designed to assist you with all of these roles. Each chapter is aimed at a specific function or problem. Unlike most books, this one does not need to be read from beginning to end. Instead, there are several ways you can get started:

- As with any other book, start with the table of contents and read what you want.
- Start with the following problem list. The chapter numbers after the problems show where you will find answers.
- As you read, you will be directed to other parts of the book for more information on related subjects.

All of this is to say that there are many roads to a good patient education program. Try whichever ones are best for you.

◘ PROBLEM LIST

1. Doctors will not
   - participate: Chapter 5
   - refer: Chapter 5
   - do what I want them to do: Chapter 5
2. Patients are not motivated: Chapters 1, 2, 4, 5, 9
3. Patients will not come: Chapter 5
4. We give the education and people don't change: Chapters 2, 4, 8, 9
5. Patients will not comply: Chapter 9
6. I do not have time: Chapter 4
7. How do we educate _____ [fill in any racial or ethnic group]? Chapters 6, 7
8. All that theory stuff does not make any sense in my "real" world: Chapter 2
9. I do not know if what I do makes a difference: Chapter 3
10. I do not have the resources to do patient education: Chapter 5
11. I do not know what to teach: Chapters 1, 4
12. How do I deal with talkative, quiet, belligerent, and other types of patients? Chapter 8
13. How do I assess learner readiness and skill level? Chapters 1, 7
14. How do I deal with groups when people come with different knowledge, skills, and interests? Chapters 1, 4
15. How can I get over administrative barriers? Chapters 1, 3, 5
16. There is not enough space for classes: Chapter 5
17. How do I work with patients from other cultures? Chapter 6
18. How do I prepare written materials? Chapter 7
19. How do I choose materials? Chapter 7
20. The marketing department wants to change my program to meet marketing needs: Chapter 5
21. How do we prepare to meet the JCAHO patient and family education requirements? Chapter 10
22. How do we get reimbursement?

How Do I Know What Patients Want and Need?
Needs Assessment

Kate Lorig

Programs that educate patients do not just happen. Rather, they are shaped by the beliefs and skills of those offering the education. All programs start with someone who believes that patients should know or do something. The program is then formed to ensure that this happens. The initial belief is the foundation of the program. The strength of the foundation, and thus of the whole program, is determined by how well the program fits the needs of those it will serve. Unfortunately, health professionals alone are usually not able to understand patient needs fully, and many programs fall short. Solid patient education programs, however, are built on carefully executed *needs assessments*.

Before I begin the discussion of how to conduct needs assessments, here is a tip on how to get others in your organization to accept the idea of doing them. Often, someone will come to you with an idea: You should make a pamphlet, put up a poster, or put together a class. The originator of the idea also knows exactly what should be written or taught. For whatever reason, you do not think this is a good idea. Rather than arguing, you can say, "It is our policy always to conduct a needs assessment or to test new materials. Let us do this with your idea and see what happens." This approach changes your role from opponent to assistant. The following are several methods of conducting needs assessments.

¤ INTERESTED-PARTY ANALYSIS

One of the most common errors in planning any new program is not considering the needs of all those involved. Although it is evident that client needs are important, we often forget the needs of the other interested parties. There are often many such persons, including the patient's family, health professionals, friends, neighbors, other service agencies, and even marketing departments. Once the general topic of a program has been determined (e.g., cancer, diabetes, AIDS, or caregiver support), it is important to make a list of all the interested parties.

The next step is to interview the key people to find out what they want from your program and how this program may affect other programs. For instance, the fund-raising branch of the organization may see the program as a source of new donors or as of special interest to a new donor community. On the other hand, they may be concerned about advertising for your program at the same time that they are pursuing another large public campaign. Furthermore, the volunteer recruiter may be overwhelmed by the need to recruit and train an additional 40 volunteers or may be overjoyed because your program will serve as a new recruiting tool. The assessment may have shown a need to provide services to a special language or cultural group. However, the agency's administration may be concerned that this would necessitate the hiring of bilingual staff, which could affect the budget. The marketing department may see your program as a way of attracting new clients.

More and more health plans are becoming interested parties. They may want patient education programs for marketing purposes or to increase patient satisfaction. In addition, they insist on evidence-based programs, programs that reduce health care utilization, or both. In planning a program, you must be very clear about the needs of the health care plan.

Other agencies in the community may also have an interest in your plans. A program to assist the adult children of aging parents may be offered by other organizations or health providers. Your agency may find itself in a turf battle that could lead to unfavorable publicity.

Finally, the needs of clients may be different from the needs of their families. Children undergoing chemotherapy may see teasing by peers as a major problem. Thus the agency could provide a teasing-inoculation program by showing parents how to help their children gain new skills and confidence to manage the teasing or by working with the children directly. However, such a program would completely ignore the needs of parents of children with cancer, who must deal with family stress and the fear of future prognosis. Because most health problems affect not only the individual but his or her family and community as well, it is important to get input from everyone before deciding the program focus.

Figure 1.1 shows a suggested interview or questionnaire format for an interested-party analysis. Remember, this format is not etched in stone; it is offered only as a guide for you to change and use as you wish. You may want to ask other questions during this same interview, regarding, for instance, the best format, place, or time for the program or how to fund the program. However, such questions are not necessary in the needs assessment

---

1. Name: _____

2. Reason for interviewing: _____ (For example, is this person a patient, a family member, an agency administrator?)

3. We are considering starting a _____ program and would be interested in your opinions. Because you are a _____, your ideas are very important.

4. Considering your position, what do you think should be the objective of the program? (For clients and their families, this question can be re-phrased as follows: When you think of _____, what do you think of?)

5. What advantages do you see in starting this program?

6. What are the disadvantages or other possible problems that you foresee?

7. How do you see yourself (your agency) participating in this program?

8. Do you have any other thoughts that you would like to share with us?

Figure 1.1. Suggested Interview/Questionnaire Format for an Interested-Party Analysis

stage and are sometimes best left until you know exactly where you are going.

In addition to the questions shown in Figure 1.1, you might ask a payer such as a health care plan or government agency, "What characteristics must this program have to be eligible for reimbursement or inclusion in the budget?" Here the trick is not to ask about *how* to get reimbursement but rather to assume that this is possible. Once some decision maker has told you what to do, all you have to do is follow instructions. Many times, this will result in a program for which you can receive reimbursement. The time to find out about reimbursement is when you are planning a program.

✪ CHECKLIST NEEDS ASSESSMENT

One of the most common forms of needs assessment is a questionnaire checklist. All you do is list a number of topics and let potential participants check off topics of interest. There are many advantages to this method. Checklists are easy to administer and to tally, and clients seldom object to them. However, checklists should not be used as the sole means of getting information. The problem is that a checklist usually reflects what professionals are ready to teach, not necessarily the interests of their patients. For example, many checklists about cardiac problems include such things as exercise, diet, and medication but fail to mention the problems of living with uncertainty. Yet we know from studies that uncertainty is usually a major concern for those patients. Why is it forgotten? Because living with uncertainty is not the central focus of any one health profession and therefore sometimes falls through the cracks.

Many checklists do include a space marked "other," but there are seldom enough similar responses in that category to make these an important program-planning consideration. Still, all is not lost. Checklists can be useful if carefully constructed. The topics to be included should come from both patients and professionals. Focus groups are sometimes useful in writing checklists (see the section on focus groups later in this chapter). Be sure not to change or misrepresent the patient-generated items—for example, by changing "living with uncertainty" to "living with frustration."

All in all, it is probably best not to rely solely on checklists. If you do, however, be sure to follow the above guidelines.

✪ SALIENT BELIEF ASSESSMENT

From psychology, we learn that human beings can have only seven or so beliefs or opinions about any one subject. These have been called *salient beliefs* (Fishbein & Ajzen, 1975; Miller, 1956). If you can identify these beliefs, you can use this knowledge as a basis for your educational efforts. Assessing salient beliefs is an especially useful strategy for the busy health care provider in one-on-one situations. A simple way of soliciting these beliefs is to ask the patient, "When you think of ____, what do you think about?" The blank can be filled in with any behavior or disease (e.g., exercise or cancer). The answers that you get will give you good insight into that person's beliefs and concerns about that particular condition or behavior.

People with arthritis most often answer the above question with "pain, disability, and depression." Knowing this, the health educator can then build a group or individual teaching program around managing pain and preventing disability. If the patient's first response is "fear," then the teaching should be aimed at determining the reason for the fear and trying to overcome it.

If the health educator wishes to establish a group program, he or she can ask a number of people with a similar condition or problem, "What do you think of when you think about ____?" They can then write as many answers to the question as they wish. These answers are then rated, with the first answer getting 10 points, the second answer 9 points, and so on. The total score is then added for each response. The responses with the highest scores are the most important for that group. Figure 1.2 provides an example of how to do this scoring.

One of the advantages of this technique is that it enables you to tailor the education to the perceptions and needs of the patients. For example, most traditional cardiac rehabilitation education does not directly address uncertainty but instead focuses on exercise, medication, and diet, which are the major concerns of health professionals working with coronary disease. These topics are all very important but may be better accepted by patients if taught in the context of being better able to live with uncertainty.

A third way of using a salient belief assessment is in presenting public lectures. Often, a health educator is asked to talk to a group about one topic or another. Because this is a one-shot song and dance, the educator generally shows a film or gives a lecture. Instead, you might start a presentation by saying something like this:

	Mary	Score	Jane	Score	Rebecca	Score
			Responses by Individual			
First response	hot flashes	10	sagging body	10	fatigue	10
Second response	growing older	9	no birth control	9	hot flashes	9
Third response	no menstruation	8	dry vagina	8	getting old	8
Fourth response	loss sex appeal	7	fatigue	7	fatigue	7

Aggregate Responses

Response	Total Score
Hot flashes	$10 + 9 = 19/3 = 6.3$
Growing older	$9 + 8 = 17/3 = 5.7$
No menstruation	$8/3 = 2.7$
Loss of sex appeal	$7/3 = 2.3$
Sagging body	$10/3 = 3.3$
No birth control	$9/3 = 3$
Dry vagina	$8/3 = 2.7$
Fatigue	$7 + 7 + 10 = 24/3 = 8.0$

Priority for Teaching	*Score*
1. Fatigue	8.0
2. Hot flashes	6.3
3. Growing old	5.7

Figure 1.2. Scoring a Salient Belief Assessment for the Question "What Do You Think of When You Think of Menopause?"

NOTE: These data are fictional; they do not necessarily represent what should be taught about menopause.

We could say lots of things about AIDS, such as what it is, who can get it, how you get it, how you prevent it, or what safe sex is. Before beginning, I want to know what you would like to know about AIDS. I will make a list, and then we will vote on how you would like me to use my time.

At this point, you ask the audience what they would like you to address. Write down all the items without comment, and then read the list. Next, give everyone two or three votes and go through the list, having the audience vote. Finally, address your talk to the top three or four items on the list.

This technique has several advantages. First, it involves the audience and lets them know that you are really interested in their input. Second, it allows you to address the issues of special interest to that group. One reason some speakers are afraid to try this technique is that they think the audience will ask something that they are not prepared to address. Of course this can happen, in which case all you have to do is say that you don't know anything about, for instance, how monoclonal antibodies affect AIDS, and go on to the next topic. Most of the time, however, the topics chosen by the audience will be well-known to you.

◘ MATRIX ASSESSMENT

This technique is especially good with a small group of no more than 15 to 20 people. It is a quick variation on nominal group process, or the Delphi process (McKillip, 1987). First, ask all participants to write a list of what they would like to learn in the class or what the major problems are that they have because of their disease. Make it clear that these lists are for reference only and will not be turned in. By having people write their individual needs first, you are assured that everyone can participate and that less popular needs will not get lost.

Create a matrix form such as that shown in Figure 1.3 (p. 9). Ask the first person to read aloud the items on his or her list, and put each item in a column heading at the top of the matrix, with the person's name as the first row heading at the side of the matrix. Then put an X by each item in his or her row. Put the name of the second person as the next row heading. Put an X by all the items that he or she names for which there are headings at the

	How to Overcome Disabilities	Choosing a Doctor	Speech Problems	Controlling High Blood Pressure	Nutrition	Smoking	Stress Management	How to Choose a Nursing Home
John	X	X	X	X				
Maria		X	X	X	X		X	
Debbie	X				X	X		
Stan	X	X		X				
Pat		X					X	
Moses	X			X		X		
Joan		X			X			
Sasha	X	X		X				
Barbara	X				X			X
Jim	X	X					X	
Total	7	7	2	5	4	2	3	1

Figure 1.3. Matrix Assessment Chart for a Class for Stroke Patients

top. Then give each new item a new column and add Xs in the appropriate columns (see Figure 1.3). Continue this process for each person in the group. After everyone has exhausted his or her list, ask if anyone wants to add any Xs anywhere on the matrix. Ideas from some of the people who spoke later may appeal to some of their peers who spoke earlier. Finally, add all the Xs in each column. The topics with the most Xs are the topics of most interest and should be emphasized. This process also allows all the participants to see how their interests fit with those of others in the group. If there is one person with very different interests, he or she may decide that this is not the appropriate group or may decide to stay without expectations of having his or her specific interests met.

◘ FOCUS GROUPS

Another way of conducting needs assessments is to get together a small number of potential clients for a focus group (Morgan, 1997). Any number from 8 to 12 is ideal (Breitrose, 1988). Smaller groups tend to inhibit conversation, and larger groups can become unwieldy. It is very important that the focus group participants be like the people you are trying to reach. Focus groups also tend to work best if the participants are similar. If you are trying to reach a very mixed audience, you might have several focus groups: one for elderly women, another for middle-aged men, and yet another for members of a specific ethnic minority community. Most focus groups should not last more than 2 hours.

The group leader should be a person unknown to the focus group participants. In addition, the leader should not have strong opinions about the topic being discussed. In fact, it is best if the leader knows very little about the topic. On the other hand, it is helpful if the leader has skills in working with groups, so that he or she can elicit opinions from all participants, and not just from one or two dominant group members. A leader who is skilled in working with groups can also ensure that all group members feel their opinions are valued.

Before the focus group is brought together, it is important to prepare the questions to be asked. Usually, three to five questions are enough. Possible questions include the following: What are the biggest problems you face with _____? What would you like to learn? What are the difficulties you have in living with someone who has _____? The secret is to be as nondirective as possible. You might start the group off with a matrix assessment and then ask the participants to discuss in more detail exactly what they would like to learn. Some people like to start a focus group with a brainstorming activity (for more on this, see Chapter 4).

You can also use a focus group to evaluate new educational material. The participants can watch a videotape or read a pamphlet and then be asked about what they liked, what they didn't like, and how they would change it. Or a focus group might be shown a potential social marketing advertisement and then be asked how they interpret the message. For example, there might be an ad with a doctor saying that when he gets back pain, he knows it is not serious and gets on with his work. The purpose of the ad is to encourage people with back pain to stay active. However, blue-collar workers may not be able to relate to such a message.

Another way to use a focus group is to follow a questionnaire. For example, you learn that stroke patients would like an exercise videotape for home use. You could then use a focus group to determine the types of exercise desired, how long the tape should be, willingness to buy the tape, and so on.

If possible, it is best to audiotape a focus group. Always have a backup tape recorder, extra batteries, and a long extension cord on hand. If anything can go wrong, it probably will. When taping, ask all participants to identify themselves each time they speak. When you cannot tape the focus group, and even if you can, it is often helpful to have someone take notes.

Focus group data are hard to interpret. As a leader or observer, you tend to hear what you want to hear. Although the ideal would be to transcribe the tape and then conduct a theme analysis, this is very labor-intensive and time-consuming. An easier method of data analysis is to have two or three impartial people read the notes or listen to the tape. Each of these judges should write down what he or she considers to be the main themes. The judges can then meet to share their thoughts on the themes and reach a consensus. If possible, one of the judges should be facing health issues similar to those of the people in the focus group. For example, people taking a self-management program listed one of the benefits as "sharing." The health professional judges interpreted this as receiving social support. However, the judge who was a patient said that he thought that people were talking about the opportunity to help others. Upon further exploration, my colleagues and I found that both views were correct, but that the "helping others" theme was stronger. Thus when we revised the program we added more opportunities for the participants to share by helping others.

Another way to use focus group data is to incorporate them into a further assessment using an incomplete block design evaluation (see the section on balanced incomplete block designs later in this chapter).

When my colleagues and I are starting a new project, we hold a series of focus groups. In the first group, we get some major themes. We ask the same question in the second group and then ask the second-group participants to discuss the major themes uncovered in the first group. We continue this process with each successive group until we are hearing no new themes and the groups become repetitive. This usually happens within four or five focus groups.

Key Message Focus Groups

The purposes of key message focus groups are to limit the amount of information that is given in patient education programs and to standardize the information. Often, patient education programs are so crammed with information that patients are overwhelmed and end up not doing anything. Another problem is that patient educators are so anxious to pass on all they know about a topic that they substitute the giving of information for the important process aspect of patient education.

Focus groups can also be held with health professionals to determine the most important messages that must be included in a program. For example, a group of arthritis educators might be asked first to list all the topics that should be included in an 8-hour program. Next, they are asked to prioritize the topics. When they reach consensus about the topics, they can be asked what three messages they want to teach about each topic, starting with the top-priority topic. This is a much more difficult task, because the tendency is to want to teach everything about every topic. As a group leader, your job is to force a discussion about the key messages. For example, the key messages about exercise might be as follows: (a) Start doing what you can do now without having more pain when you finish than before you start, (b) exercise 4-5 days a week, and (c) add to your exercise program by 10%-20% per week until you are exercising 20 to 30 minutes a week—remember that you don't have to do all your exercise at one time.

¤ STRUCTURED AND SEMISTRUCTURED INTERVIEWS

Another way of conducting needs assessments is through an interview. For this, you make an interview format similar to that shown in Figure 1.4. A group of people like those you are trying to reach are all interviewed using the same format. These interviews can be done in person or by phone. Our experience suggests that phone interviews are usually just as effective as face-to-face interviews and are much more efficient. In addition, the phone allows you to interview people you could not reach in person. Of course, if the people you wish to reach do not have phones, face-to-face interviews are necessary. Public opinion polls are good examples of the use of structured interviews.

---

1. When you think of diabetes, what do you think of? (Note: This is a "salient belief" question.)
2. What are your greatest problems in living with diabetes?
3. Would you attend a 6-week class on diabetes?

   If yes:

       3a. Where should it be held?

       3b. What times are best for you?

       3c. What topics would you like covered?

   If no:

       3d. How would you like to learn about diabetes?
4. What would you like to know about diabetes?
5. What else about your diabetes would you like to tell us?

Figure 1.4. Sample Semistructured Interview

Structured interviews are good in that, like checklists, they are easy to administer and tally. In addition, you have the opportunity to clarify anything you do not understand. The disadvantage, as with checklists, is that you will never discover concerns that the interview does not cover. One way to get around this is by adding some open-ended or semistructured questions to your structured interview. If you do this, the open-ended questions should come before the structured questions. This helps prevent getting the answers that the participants think you want to hear.

After you have completed your interviews, you can analyze the responses using the qualitative evaluation technique discussed in Chapter 3.

✪ BALANCED INCOMPLETE BLOCK DESIGN

Many of the needs assessment techniques discussed above—salient belief assessments, focus groups, and semistructured interviews—result in data that are somewhat hard to interpret.

The use of an incomplete block design analysis helps solve this problem. Although this second-level assessment makes the process more complex, it results in data that are prioritized so that you know not only the priority but also the strength of the priority. For important patient education projects, the resulting information is well worth the effort.

The balanced incomplete block design technique offers a very efficient means of ranking items in a list through a series of forced comparisons. It produces a weighted ranking that shows the relative importance of each item in the list. It allows comparison of content and process items.

In the technique, all items are compared with one another using several sets of items (typically three or four per set). Subjects are asked to order each set from most to least (e.g., *most important* to *least important*). The rank order is obtained through the summing of the ranks assigned to each item.

The steps of doing a balanced incomplete block design study are as follows:

1. *List items.* List items to be ranked. This list is developed from the themes that emerged from your focus group or semistructured interviews. Typically, two or three people read the transcript of the focus group or interviews and then agree on themes. Figure 1.5 lists seven elements in a patient education program.

2. *Select design.* Count the number of items in your list and select the appropriate block design by using Figure 1.7. Each design consists of a series of questions in which the respondent is asked to rank order three or four items from the list in terms of their importance. In our sample list in Figure 1.5, there are seven items, so we will use Design A. If the number of items in your list is not given in Figure 1.7, you will have to construct your own block design (see Weller & Romney, 1988).

3. *Create form.* Create a form by using the block design and your list of items. The form should contain instructions and a series of questions that group items according to the block design. See

1. Exercise	Starting an exercise program; learning how to monitor exercise
2. Medication	Proper use of medications
3. Symptom management	Using the mind for symptom management (e.g., relaxation, visualization)
4. Communicating with doctors	Improving interactions with doctors and other health professionals
5. Problem solving	Learning to identify problems and to use techniques such as brainstorming to solve problems
6. Self-confidence	Gaining self-confidence about being able to manage symptoms
7. Sharing	Sharing experiences with other students and learning from them

Figure 1.5. Sample List for Block Design: Elements in Chronic Disease Self-Management Course

SOURCE: Campbell, Sengupta, Santos, and Lorig (1995).

Figure 1.6 for our sample form. Our series of questions is constructed from our item list and Design A. For example, the first question asks the respondent to rank order Items 1, 2, and 4.

4. *Administer form.* This can be done either orally or in writing. We recommend the written form. For suggestions on the oral form, see Weller and Romney (1988).

5. *Tabulate results.* Tabulate results by summing ranks assigned to each item. To find the mean, divide the sum by the number of respondents. One method of tabulation is shown in Figure 1.8.

One note of caution about conducting needs assessments: If you already know what you are going to do and have no intention of changing, do not conduct a needs assessment. Nothing makes people angrier than being asked their opinions and then having those opinions ignored.

Chronic Disease Self-Management Assessment

NAME _____

DATE _____

We are interested in finding out how you rate the relative importance of various aspects of the proposed course. For the sets numbered 1 to 7 below, please mark each of the three items from most important (1) to least important (3).

As an example, consider ranking the colors blue, red, and green. If your favorite color among this group is red, you would place a "1" in the blank next to "Red" (see below). If your second favorite is green, you would place a "2" next to "Green" and a "3" next to Blue."

___ Blue	_1_ Red	___ Green

1. ___ Exercise	___ Medication	___ Communicating with doctors
2. ___ Medication	___ Symptom management	___ Problem solving
3. ___ Symptom management	___ Communicating with doctors	___ Self-confidence
4. ___ Communicating with doctors	___ Problem solving	___ Sharing
5. ___ Problem solving	___ Self-confidence	___ Exercise
6. ___ Self-confidence	___ Sharing	___ Medication
7. ___ Sharing	___ Exercise	___ Symptom management

Figure 1.6. Sample Needs Assessment Form Using Block Design
SOURCE: Campbell et al. (1995).

◘ EPI INFO: A TOOL FOR DATA ANALYSIS

The preparation and analysis of data can be made much easier by the use of a public-domain software product called Epi Info. This program was written at the Centers for Disease Control in

Design A, for 7 Items	Design C, for 13 Items
1. Items 1, 2, 4	1. Items 1, 4, 5, 12
2. Items 2, 3, 5	2. Items 2, 5, 6, 13
3. Items 3, 4, 6	3. Items 3, 6, 7, 1
4. Items 4, 5, 7	4. Items 4, 7, 8, 2
5. Items 5, 6, 1	5. Items 5, 8, 9, 3
6. Items 6, 7, 2	6. Items 6, 9, 10, 4
7. Items 7, 1, 3	7. Items 7, 10, 11, 5
	8. Items 8, 11, 12, 6
Design B, for 9 Items	9. Items 9, 12, 13, 7
1. Items 1, 2, 3	10. Items 10, 13, 1, 8
2. Items 4, 5, 6	11. Items 11, 1, 2, 9
3. Items 7, 8, 9	12. Items 12, 2, 3, 10
4. Items 1, 4, 7	13. Items 13, 3, 4, 11
5. Items 2, 5, 8	
6. Items 3, 6, 9	
7. Items 1, 5, 9	
8. Items 2, 6, 7	
9. Items 3, 4, 8	
10. Items 1, 6, 8	
11. Items 2, 4, 9	
12. Items 3, 5, 7	

Figure 1.7. Some Balanced Incomplete Block Designs

SOURCE: Campbell et al. (1995).

Atlanta, Georgia, and was originally intended for use by public health officials investigating outbreaks of infectious disease. Despite its specialized beginnings, Epi Info is a versatile tool for the preparation of questionnaires of all kinds. Answers to questions can be entered on the computer and automatically added to a database. The resulting information can be analyzed with a variety of statistical tests and can be printed out in tabular or graphical form.

Category	1	2	3	Sum	N	Score
1. Exercise	111	11	1	10	6	1.6
2. Medication						
3. Symptom management						
4. Communication with doctors						
5. Problem solving						
6. Self-confidence						
7. Sharing						

Figure 1.8. Ranking Study Tally Sheet
SOURCE: Campbell et al. (1995).

Epi Info includes its own word processor, but questions can be prepared using standard office word-processing programs and transferred to Epi Info. Questionnaire data can be exported to other spreadsheet, database, or statistical analysis programs (such as SPSS).

Perhaps the best thing about Epi Info is that it is inexpensive. The latest version (Epi Info 6) costs about $35 and can be ordered from USD Inc. at 2156-D West Park Court, Stone Mountain, GA 30087; phone (404) 469-4098; World Wide Web address http://www.cdc.gov/epo/epi/epiinfo.htm. One drawback is that Epi Info is currently available only for IBM-compatible computers.

In this chapter I have addressed several ways of conducting needs assessments. There are also many other ways, including surveys, attitude-behavior-belief scales, and sampling. There is no one right or wrong way. Rather, you should use the method or methods that best fit your situation and that will give you the information you need.

Patient education is not a science; there is no exact formula. It is an art, and thus it is up to you to mix and match methods to achieve the best program for your situation.

▣ BIBLIOGRAPHY

Breitrose, P. (1988). *Focus groups—When and how to use them: A practical guide.* Stanford, CA: Stanford University, Health Promotion Resource Center.

Campbell, B. F., Sengupta, F., Santos, C., & Lorig, K. (1995). Balanced incomplete block design: Description, case study, and implications for practice. *Health Education Quarterly, 22,* 201-210.

Fishbein, M., & Ajzen, I. (1975). *Belief, attitude, intention, and behavior: An introduction to theory and research.* Reading, MA: Addison-Wesley.

McKillip, J. (1987). *Need analysis: Tools for the human services and education.* Newbury Park, CA: Sage.

Miller, G. A. (1956). The magical number seven, plus or minus two: Some limits on our capacity for processing information. *Psychological Review, 63,* 81-87.

Morgan, D. L. (1997). *Focus groups as qualitative research* (2nd ed.). Thousand Oaks, CA: Sage.

Weller, S., & Romney, A. K. (1988). *Systematic data collection.* Newbury Park, CA: Sage.

2

What Do We Know About What Works?
The Role of Theory in Patient Education

Thomas R. Prohaska
Kate Lorig

Twenty years ago, patient education was largely atheoretical. That is, we did not have strong theories or much evidence that their use made much difference. Today, all that has changed. Although there is still much work to be done, it is irresponsible to plan a patient education program that is not based on one or more theories. This chapter discusses some of the theories most commonly used in developing patient education programs.

How do we decide what should be included in a good program of patient education? What components of the program are needed to make significant and long-lasting changes in patients' attitudes, beliefs and behaviors, health, and health care utilization? With all the possible patient education interventions that exist, how do you know which programs (or components of programs) are best for your patient population, your setting, your targeted health outcomes? Having an understanding of theories and models of behavior change can provide you with a basis for making informed decisions on how to put together effective interventions in patient education. This chapter focuses on a variety of theories and models of behavior change commonly used in patient education, and the basic components of these models and theories are discussed. Our goal is to provide sufficient background on these theories so that you can make use of them in the development of patient education programs.

It is common for practitioners to feel that the application of theory has limited utility in the design and implementation of patient education programs. The use of theory and models is fundamental to the research process, and it is just as important to practitioners. In fact, Kurt Lewin, the father of health education theory, is reported to have said, "There is nothing so practical as a good theory." The value of a theory or model of behavior change can be measured according to how well its components lead to the design of an efficient and effective patient education program that takes into account the patient population, setting, and targeted health outcomes.

A theory's utility to practitioners is frequently determined by its commonsense application to intended patient education activities. If a particular theory or model is compatible with your personal experience or makes intuitive sense (i.e., it has face validity), then it is likely that you will incorporate it into the program. However, this perspective can limit program development by leading to a focus on a favorite model or theoretical perspective that may not be effective for the individual behavior in question. In reality, no one theory or model fits all the circumstances you will encounter in your practice. The more comfortable you can become with multiple theories and models, the more likely it is that you will be able to identify the best possible model or, more likely, components of multiple theories and models to guide your patient education intervention.

I have chosen the models and theories discussed in this chapter based on two criteria. First, the theories addressed here have been widely applied across a variety of populations, settings, and target behaviors and have been found generally to work well in health promotion interventions and patient education programs. Second, these theories and models have a level of overlap and yet individual uniqueness that you may find of value when you consider them as guides to program development. For example, all of the models and theories covered in this chapter assume that the patient's behavior is a result of rational cognitive decisions based on a desire to avoid illness and disability. One theory stresses the role and influence of significant other persons (social norms) in determining the patient's intentions for a course of action (theory of reasoned action); another model includes a component on the patient's perception of his or her ability to perform the behavior (self-efficacy) and the expected results (outcome efficacy) from performing the behavior (social learning theory). Determining which models or theories to select for your patient education program is a matter of identifying which theory components best address the population and fit the targeted behaviors and the setting under which the program will be implemented. Some of the strengths and weaknesses of the various models and theories are also discussed below, as well as when it is best to use particular ones.

✪ RATIONAL BEHAVIORAL RISK FACTORS AND DISEASE MANAGEMENT

McElroy and Crump (1994) discuss a major transition in health and health care in the United States from a focus on acute and infectious diseases to a focus on chronic diseases as the leading causes of death and disability. Chronic illnesses such as heart disease, lung disease, cancer, and stroke are major causes of death in the United States; the major causes of disability also include chronic illnesses such as arthritis, hypertension, and diabetes. We now recognize that many of the risk factors associated with the onset and development of these chronic illnesses are behavioral in nature. McGinnis and Foege (1993) found that approximately half of all deaths that occurred among U.S. residents in 1990 could be attributed to identifiable external factors, including behavioral health risk factors of tobacco use, diet, physical inactivity, and use of alcohol. They conclude that tobacco use accounts for approximately 400,000 deaths each year in the United States, whereas poor diet and sedentary activity account for at least 300,000 deaths each year. It is important to note that these same factors contribute to the heavy burden of most chronic diseases. This increase in chronic illness and the understanding of the role of self-management and behavioral risk factors has led to the current emphasis on patient education.

Self-care practices and behavioral risk factors not only contribute to the onset of chronic illnesses but can have major impacts on disability associated with chronic illness. Even if persons have one or more chronic illnesses, they may not have to experience increases in disability or a deterioration in their quality of life. Kaplan (1997) makes this point in an illustration of the various levels of patient education interventions (see Figure 2.1). The optimal point for education is in primary prevention (Figure 2.1, part a). This is education to prevent the development of a specific chronic illness and is preferable to efforts to reduce the impact of the illness once it has developed. Primary prevention is not only important for those who are free of disease; it is also meaningful for preventing or delaying the onset of specific chronic conditions in persons who may currently have other chronic illnesses. Patients with arthritis or diabetes may find primary prevention for cardiovascular disease just as valuable as may those without chronic illnesses. Chronic illnesses are gradual in their onset, and diseases may be present at a subclinical level. Patient education is important for some individuals whose conditions are at the subclinical stage so that the progression rate of their chronic disease to a more advanced, clearly clinically detectable state of the chronic illness may be slowed (Figure 2.1, part b). Education to reduce hypertension and cholesterol levels is an example. Patient education is important at this point in order to slow down the disease progression to prevent the onset of disability. Programs directed at this level are frequently viewed as secondary prevention (Figure 2.1, part c). At some point, disease seriously affects the patient's quality of life, leading to limitations in mobility, changes in role functioning, and reduced social interactions (Figure 2.1, part d). Patient education efforts to avoid or lessen major disability, loss of important roles, and premature death are classically termed tertiary prevention (Figure 2.1, part e). Patient education is important at all phases of primary, secondary, and tertiary prevention.

The levels displayed in Figure 2.1 may also be used to help identify reasonable outcomes of patient education at various levels of primary, secondary, and tertiary prevention. For example, a patient education program at the primary prevention level may have as its goal improved eating habits or an exercise program for older adults to promote health and to help prevent or delay a number of chronic illnesses. Secondary patient education might focus on early detection of breast cancer or hypertension. Tertiary patient education programs might focus on self-management for persons with arthritis, diabetes, or other identified diseases in order to prevent or slow disability and loss of important life roles.

All forms of prevention and patient education share the overall goal of promoting active life expectancy and compression of morbidity rather than simply extending average life expectancy. The agenda of patient education is to maximize the

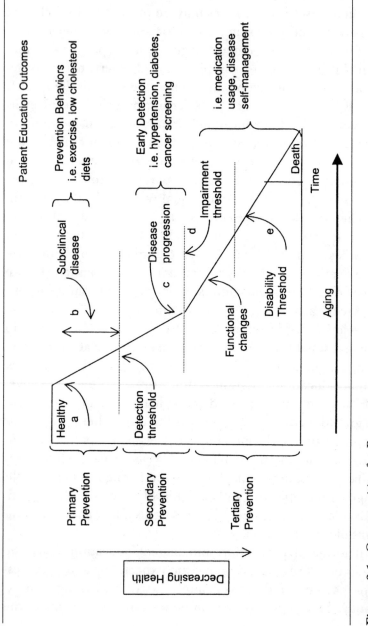

Figure 2.1. Opportunities for Prevention

SOURCE: Based on Kaplan (1997).

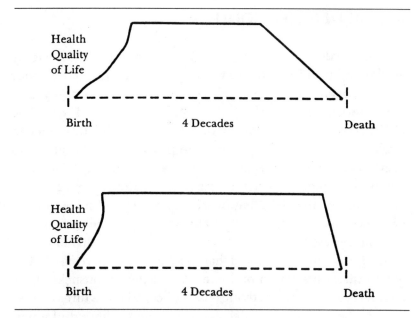

Figure 2.2. Natural "Life History" of Morbidity at Present and Projected as a Goal of Health Education

amount of time that persons experience healthy lives, with minimal time spent experiencing morbidity. Compression of morbidity (Fries & Crapo, 1981) assumes that improvements in healthy ways of living and proper self-care for chronic illnesses can postpone the onset of major disability until nearer the end of life and thereby increase the amount of time persons are free of disability. This is often referred to as an *increase in active life expectancy* or *compression of morbidity*. Figure 2.2 illustrates compression of morbidity. Stated simply, a primary objective of patient education is not to add years to life but rather to add life to years. Given our current knowledge about the role of behavioral risk factors in contributing to morbidity and mortality, it makes sense that patient education would focus on methods for behavior change and the role of theory and models in contributing to behavior change and maintaining or improving health status.

▲ ⌐EALTH BELIEF MODEL

The health belief model (HBM) is one of the most widely used theoretical frameworks for understanding health behavior and has been used extensively in patient education programs and interventions (Becker, 1974; Janz & Becker, 1984). The HBM grew out of an effort by the U.S. Public Health service to explain the failure of populations to participate in programs to prevent or detect disease, such as the lack of participation in tuberculosis screening programs (secondary prevention). Since its development, the HBM has been applied beyond screening behaviors to a variety of health behaviors, illness behaviors, and chronic disease management. The model assumes that individuals desire to avoid illness and that specific actions in response to a health threat are based on beliefs about the seriousness of the health threat and the activities used to combat the threat.

The health belief model states that the likelihood of a person's taking action in response to a health threat is dependent on that person's beliefs and perceptions, including his or her perceived susceptibility to the illness, perceived severity or consequences of the illness, expectancies of benefits and barriers associated with taking the course of action (e.g., changing diet, exercising regularly, getting a mammogram), and any cues to action that trigger the action. *Perceived susceptibility* refers to the odds of contracting the illness or health risk. In general, if persons with hypertension believe that they are at increased risk for other chronic illnesses, they are more likely to pursue a course of action that will minimize the risk. It is important to uncover the patient's perception of his or her own risk rather than of risk in general, because it is very common for an individual to believe that his or her risk for adverse health is lower than that of the general public. One way of doing this is to ask patients what they are afraid may happen as a result of their disease. *Perceived severity* relates to the individual's beliefs about the consequences of the disease and of not taking the recommended actions to minimize the threat. For example, does the individual believe that AIDS is still a life-threatening disease? In general, the greater the perceived severity of the disease and the eventual consequences of not taking appropriate action, the greater the likelihood that the person will perform the desired actions. Together, the perceived susceptibility and severity of the disease combine to produce an overall perceived threat of the disease. That is, when susceptibility and severity are high, motivation to perform the desired behavior change is high. However, if the person believes his or her own susceptibility or severity to be low, then the likelihood of behavior change is reduced. For example, most people would agree that HIV infection and AIDS are very serious. If, however, they feel their individual chances of becoming infected are low, they are less likely to take preventive actions such as limiting sexual partners and using condoms.

Even though a patient believes that his or her threat of disease is high, behavior change must also consider the person's beliefs about the effectiveness of the targeted behaviors in reducing the disease threat. That is, the patient will subjectively evaluate the *benefits and barriers* involved in performing the particular health action. Each behavior has benefits and barriers associated with it. These vary considerably from behavior to behavior, even in the same disease. For example, in a diabetes education program, the same patient may exhibit different levels of behavior change for medication management, physical activity, and dietary changes. The person with diabetes may feel that diabetes is a serious health problem and that all three behaviors are important. He or she may take appropriate medication and participate in recommended exercise but not change his or her diet because of perceived barriers to dietary change. Patient compliance with dietary, physical activity, and medication self-management recommendations may differ considerably because of differences in perceived sustained effort (barriers) and potential impact on the course of the disease (benefits) in the context of overall quality of life (benefits and barriers). Although it is not usually discussed within the health belief model, it is also important to examine the time frame during which the patient can expect to see these benefits. For example, if a person with chronic obstructive pulmonary disease participates in an exercise program and expects to see major improvement in a short period of time, he or she may become frustrated with the apparent lack of progress and drop out of the program. Another example is the person with arthritis who stops taking prescribed medication when there is no noticeable pain relief in 48 hours. (Many arthritis medications take from a week to several months to affect pain.) A key to addressing benefits properly in a patient education program is to identify realistic outcomes of the behavior that are meaningful to the participant and that are based on an accurate time frame. This could be as simple as telling patients when to expect results from the medications they are taking.

Cues to action, another component of the HBM, can be thought of as including any event or stimulus that triggers patients to perform the targeted behaviors. The rationale for this construct is that patients are more likely to perform the desired behaviors when they are reminded or have cues to perform the behavior. For example, a patient who receives an appointment reminder card from his or her dentist may be more likely to keep the appointment. A cue to action may also be internal, such as experiencing pain. However, we cannot manipulate internal cues, and it is common for symptoms of chronic illnesses to be associated with normal aging, resulting in a tendency not to respond. We can also help patients reinterpret these internal cues (see the discussion of self-efficacy below). Health behavior interventions frequently include some form of a cue to action as part of the program, such as use of a log or notes to oneself. The cues given by symptoms can be used to form educational messages, such as "You should not have more pain after exercising than before you start, but exercise may not be pain free" or "If you are short of breath, slow down; if shortness of breath continues, stop and take your medication."

The HBM also recognizes the importance of sociodemographic characteristics (e.g., age, ethnicity, gender, sexual orientation, socioeconomic status) of the person that may influence the beliefs and perceptions components of the model. Members of different demographic groups differ in their perceptions and attitudes and in their propensity to perform specific health behaviors, including health screening (e.g., mammograms, hypertension screening), health promotion behaviors (e.g., exercise, smoking cessation, alcohol consumption), and health protective behaviors (e.g., getting flu shots). As a result, patient education programs based on the HBM may be effective for some behaviors but may need to be modified for population subgroups. It is important to understand how various cultural and demographic groups differ in terms of attitudes and perceptions of the illness, the behavior, and their own risk. Even here, you need to be careful. As discussed in Chapter 6, there are often as many differences within groups as there are across groups.

The HBM provides an excellent road map for identifying the key informational components of a patient education program. When patients are not knowledgeable about their risk profiles for a specific health threat, have unrealistic beliefs concerning their own susceptibilities, underestimate the severity of the health threat, or have inappropriate beliefs about the barriers and benefits of a course of action, the HBM can provide a framework to address those knowledge gaps. It is an excellent model for ensuring that you have covered many of the essential components of an educational message in a comprehensive manner. If you have adequately addressed all of the components of the HBM, the patient should have a basic understanding of the health threat and the importance of adhering to recommended regimes.

However, it must be noted that although knowledge is necessary for behavior change, it is generally not sufficient. Health behavior interventions based solely on the health belief model will frequently demonstrate only modest improvements. Patients may correctly perceive their susceptibility and the severity of the health threat and the consequences of performing or not performing the activities. They may also have been exposed to a cue to action and yet still not be performing the behaviors. They may not participate in or adhere to the new behaviors if they do not feel capable of performing the targeted activities. One reason for this is that they may not feel that they have the necessary skills or capability to perform the behaviors. Although the concept of perceived capability and self-confidence in performing behaviors has recently been added to the HBM, a better model that more fully addresses this concept is Albert Bandura's social cognitive theory, which is described below.

¤ SOCIAL COGNITIVE THEORY

According to Bandura's social cognitive theory (also referred to as *social learning theory;* see Bandura, 1997; Bandura & Strunk, 1981; Clark & Dodge, 1999), an individual's perceptions of his or her ability to perform an action (self-efficacy) and his or her expectations that the behavior will have a desirable result (outcome efficacy) are important mediators of performance. Social cognitive theory states that behavior change is a result of setting personal goals based on self-efficacy expectations for performing the behavior and of the outcome expectations associated with the results of engaging in the behavior. If a person believes that he or she is capable of performing a behavior and also believes that the behavior will lead to desired outcomes, the person will be more likely to perform the behavior. Let us examine these concepts more closely.

Self-Efficacy Expectations

Self-efficacy refers to a person's judgments about ability to monitor, plan, and carry out a specific behavior. Self-efficacy is based on the recognition that if individuals are to try a behavior, they must first believe that they have the necessary skills to engage in that behavior. If an individual does not *believe* that he or she is capable of performing the behavior, that person will have no incentive to do so, even if he or she actually is capable. In short, when people believe they can do something, they probably can; when they do not believe they can do something, they probably will not try. Self-efficacy is part of a reciprocal process resulting from an interaction among personal, behavioral, and environmental factors that determines behavior. It is reciprocal in that perceptions of self-efficacy influence behavior change and in that the observation of one's own behavior influences perceptions of self-efficacy. For example, if a person with diabetes thinks that he or she can eat some protein for breakfast, that person may try some yogurt, find that it helps keep his or her energy up, and thus be more sure (increase his or her self-efficacy) that he or she will eat some protein every morning. Perceived capacity to perform a behavior is dependent on the particular situation or context for the behavior, and self-efficacy for a specific behavior can vary from situation to situation. For example, a person with diabetes may feel quite capable of adhering to medical dietary recommendations when eating at home but may feel incapable, or nonefficacious, when it comes to staying within dietary recommendations while traveling or when eating in restaurants.

Perceptions of self-efficacy are particularly important for complex activities and long-term changes in behavior. These are frequently the objectives of patient education programs. For example, starting and maintaining an aerobic exercise program after a heart attack will require an individual to perceive that he or she is capable of performing the exercise activities without harm. In addition, the person must believe that exercise participation will lead to desired outcomes, such as prevention of a subsequent heart attack. Perceived self-efficacy may be lower in persons with limited experience with a behavior, such as those newly diagnosed with diabetes who have no experience with monitoring their blood sugar level or with self-injecting insulin. Perceptions of self-efficacy may also be lower in individuals who have experienced multiple failed attempts at the behavior as well as in those who are experiencing a loss of physical or mental abilities.

There are four major methods for developing and enhancing efficacy expectations; these involve (a) performance accomplishments, (b) vicarious experience or modeling, (c) verbal persuasion, and (d) interpretation of physiological state. The first of these, performance accomplishments, may be the most direct and influential way to enhance self-efficacy in that learning is acquired through personal experience with actually performing the tasks. Patient education programs focusing on skills mastery frequently break down the desired tasks into smaller, more manageable tasks. People first perform the easier tasks, the ones they are sure they can perform. By attending to and succeeding with the immediate tasks, people develop a sense of competence and self-efficacy for completing the more difficult tasks. In short, self-motivation is achieved faster and more effectively through the setting and accomplishment of proximal, short-term goals than through the setting of distal, long-term goals (Bandura & Strunk, 1981). For example, a person starting an exercise program may be asked to walk for however long he or she can now walk (even if it is only 5 minutes) and to do this four times a week. When the individual has successfully accomplished this, the program can be added to slowly. (In the protocol that appears in Appendix 4B in Chapter 4, performance accomplishments are achieved through action planning.)

Single-task repetition at each step enhances self-efficacy and skills mastery. As each subgoal is achieved, the person should repeatedly perform the task before going on to the next-least-difficult task. This will increase self-confidence and task persistence and provide a foundation of success and mastery for the next, slightly more difficult task. For example, it is probably unrealistic to expect a person newly diagnosed with diabetes to feel competent at and capable of self-injecting insulin. Rather than merely telling that person how to self-inject, the technique of skills mastery would suggest that the self-injection process be divided into subtasks ranging from the easiest to the most difficult (e.g., thoroughly cleaning the skin for needle penetration, correctly holding the syringe, drawing the correct amount of insulin, removing air bubbles, needle injection into an object, self-injection), and providing opportunities for repeated practice at each step prior to going on to the next. Practice at each step and combination of the steps will enhance self-efficacy for the entire process. When a health educator is helping a patient with skills mastery, it is very important that the patient succeed at each step. If there is a failure, patient and educator should discuss it, analyze the problem, and change the expected skill performance so that the patient can achieve success.

　　Another method of enhancing self-efficacy is through modeling—that is, by having the patient observe others who appear to be similar. This method is particularly useful for groups of persons dealing with the same illness or chronic condition. When patients believe that they are among others who are very similar to them, with the same challenges, and they see one of those others successfully perform a behavior, they are very likely to think, "If that person can do it, maybe I can do it, too." For example, the Save Our Sisters Project relied on minority women who had participated in mammography screening to go into the community and persuade other women to get mammograms (Eng, 1993). This is learning through vicarious experience. A person who succeeds at the task serves as a model for others.

　　The key to choosing a good model to demonstrate the behavior is to be realistic. You want the model to be viewed as someone who is no different from the other patients in the program. A good source for such role models is the population of successful participants who have taken part in past patient education programs. Those who have participated in previous programs can relate to the realities of the disease and the challenges of performing the behavior. Be careful not to pick a "supermodel," someone who has succeeded against all odds, such as the amputee who is a champion race walker. Such people are good for inspiration but may well be seen by the ordinary patient as doing the impossible.

Another way of modeling is to be sure that the illustrations in books and pamphlets represent patients' reality. For example, when showing pictures of exercises, you should make sure not only that the models represent various ethnic groups, but that they reflect different body shapes and ages. Informal modeling can be done through the placement of patients in the hospital: Someone about to undergo bypass surgery can be placed in a room with someone about to go home after the same kind of surgery. Finally, modeling can be used in program publicity materials in which past participants tell their stories or offer brief remarks.

Persuasion is the third common and effective method of enhancing efficacy expectations. The content of the message in verbal persuasion can include basic factual information stressing the importance of performing the behavior, use of fear to persuade the person to comply, or encouragement and support for the person to do the behavior.

It is usually better to ask patients to do just slightly more than they are doing now. For example, do not say, "You need to lose 80 pounds"; rather, say, "What do you think you could do to lose 3-4 pounds in the next month?" Finally, family members, friends, and other groups are very useful in supplying persuasion. If "everyone" is exercising or not smoking, it is easier for your patient to change his or her behavior.

Interpretation of physiological states is the fourth method for enhancing self-efficacy. Not only do most diseases have symptoms, but most new behaviors bring about a degree of emotional arousal and physiological change. For example, persons trying to quit smoking may expect withdrawal symptoms, and persons with arthritis may expect and experience pain when exercising. Addressing the meaning of these symptoms and physiological states can influence self-efficacy. In the example of aerobic exercise for older adults, low perceptions of self-efficacy may be the result of fear of pain that they consider medically dangerous if they perform the exercise. This is reinforced by the experience of physical fatigue and increased "heart pounding" with physical activity. If you explain that the pain may be due to weak, stressed muscles and that exercise will help to remedy that problem, you may lessen their fear of exercise.

In addition, showing older adults how to monitor their heart rate and their own rate of perceived exertion using the Borg Scale can lead to a greater sense of confidence for the individual that no harm is occurring (Borg, 1982). (The Borg Scale asks a person to rate his or her exertion on a scale of 0 to 10, with 0 being no exertion and 10 being very heavy exertion. A range of 3-5 is considered safe aerobic activity.) This leads to a greater sense of self-efficacy for participating in exercise activities.

It may seem obvious to say that if people perform specific behaviors, they will feel capable of doing those behaviors. However, once patients perform the desired behaviors, it becomes important to ensure that they are correctly monitoring the behaviors and are attributing their performance to their capabilities. This is especially true of patient education behaviors that may include multiple and complex tasks. People may feel that they are not capable of continuing the tasks and may assume that their past performance was luck or chance and is not likely to continue, or that they simply cannot remember all aspects of the patient education program. Self-efficacy theory suggests that proper appraisal of efficacy information should be incorporated into patient education programs.

There are a number of ways you can provide opportunities for patients to appraise their performance properly, resulting in increased perceptions of self-efficacy for the behavior. Teaching a patient proper self-monitoring and proper interpretation of the behavior is one such way. For example, persons with hypertension, stroke, or cardiovascular problems may show low self-efficacy for performing regular exercise. Part of their apprehension may stem from concern that if they do not exercise properly, they may have another illness episode (stroke, heart attack). However, teaching such patients that not exercising is more dangerous than exercising and helping them to monitor their own heart rate and to evaluate their rate of perceived exertion accurately (on the Borg Scale) can provide them with the necessary feedback they need to understand that their exercise level is correct and safe. Although this concept can overlap with the concept of outcome expectations (to be discussed next), techniques to ensure proper appraisal of efficacy information are aimed at facilitating interpretations of behavior into increases in perceptions of self-efficacy for the behavior; they are not necessarily the desired outcomes for the person.

Outcome Expectations

Once a patient is performing the desired behaviors, the objective is to keep him or her performing those behaviors. Outcome expectations, another component of the self-efficacy model, are related to this issue. Examples of outcome expectations are being strong enough to go up 15 steps to attend a friend's party and being able to take a desired trip. In general, a person is more likely to continue to perform a behavior if the behavior leads to a desired outcome. People have expectations as to the benefits of participation in the behavior program. They also have timelines for when they expect to see these results. It is important that their expectations be realistic. Unrealistic goals are often a direct path to failure. There is a greater chance that patients will not continue to participate in the program if they do not see progress toward their goals. Thus it is often helpful to break big goals into doable weekly steps or action plans (see Chapter 4). If a person's goals and timeline are unrealistic, you can help him or her to set new goals or to develop a new time frame.

¤ THEORY OF REASONED ACTION/ PLANNED BEHAVIOR

Like the other theories discussed in this chapter, the theory of reasoned action (TRA) assumes that people usually behave in a rational manner and that behavior is under the individual's control (Ajzen & Fishbein, 1980). Unlike social cognitive theory, the TRA has a greater application for behaviors that do not require skills building. The theory of reasoned action states that performance of a behavior is largely dependent on the individual's choice to perform that behavior. Therefore, the individual's *intention* to perform the behavior is the deciding factor in whether or not the behavior is performed. That is, intention is assumed to be highly related to behavior (Ajzen, 1988).

Intention, in turn, is determined by two basic characteristics: the individual's attitudes about the behavior and subjective norms. Attitudes toward the behavior are the person's positive and negative evaluations about performing the behavior. Subjective norms are the person's *beliefs* about how people important to the person feel about the behavior and how motivated the person is to comply with the wishes of those significant others. The assumption in the TRA is that the person is likely to perform the desired behavior when he or she has a positive view of the behavior, assumes that significant others (e.g., family and friends) want him or her to perform the behavior, and is motivated to comply.

The influence of attitudes in the theory of reasoned action is similar to perceptions of barriers and benefits in performing the behavior found in the health belief model. The person perceives both positive and negative consequences of performing and not performing the behavior and weighs these perceptions to determine his or her intention to perform the behavior. The attitude toward the behavior is similar to that in Bandura's social cognitive theory in that the belief can be linked with some valued outcome of the behavior (outcome expectations). Subjective norms share characteristics with the concept of social support for behaviors. When people believe that persons important to them have expectations that they will perform, and when they are motivated to comply with these expectations, the greater will be their intention to perform. For some behaviors, the subjective norms are a more important determinant of intention; for other behaviors, it is the attitude toward the behavior that is crucial. The TRA also assumes that the strength of the intention is directly proportional to the strength of the two components: attitudes toward the behavior and subjective norms.

The TRA specifies the factors that maximize the association between intention and behavior. First, the shorter the time interval between the statement of intention and the performance of the behavior, the greater the association. This makes intuitive sense, in that the longer the time between intention and behavior, the greater the probability that other intervening factors may influence the behavior. Second, the more specific the behavioral intention, the greater the likelihood of compliance with the behavior later. For example, you are far more likely to get a patient to commit to an intention to change his or her salt intake by starting with not using table salt tomorrow than by trying to get the patient to commit to change his or her entire diet sometime soon.

Here, action planning can be applied (see the script in Appendix 4B). This aspect of the TRA is somewhat analogous to recommendations based in social cognitive theory to start with specific tasks that the person knows he or she can perform, rather than starting skills mastery with the more difficult tasks. The theory of reasoned action is also similar to social cognitive theory in that greater confidence in intention to do the behavior is associated with a greater likelihood of behavior performance.

The theory of reasoned action is particularly useful for recognizing the social nature of behavior. Patient education programs that target behaviors that are influenced by social interactions and social influences can benefit from the social norms component of the TRA. For example, dietary behavior is highly influenced by family and friends. It is difficult to change a person's eating habits when he or she perceives little support from family for the changes. This theory also points to a general strategy for intervening in attitudes toward a behavior. The TRA states that attitudes (positive and negative evaluations) toward a behavior are additive. For example, a person may believe that changing to foods lower in fat that help lower HDL cholesterol might "reduce my chances of a heart attack," "help me lose weight and feel better," "result in boring meals," "require a lot of effort," and other outcome evaluations. Changing intention and ultimately behavior is a matter of addressing each salient outcome to assure that the advantages outweigh the disadvantages. Thus it is important to spend education time in problem solving and overcoming barriers.

Unfortunately, the theory of reasoned action is limited in that not all behaviors are simply a matter of the individual's choice. As noted in the discussion of social cognitive theory, some behaviors, at least initially, are not under the individual's control. Also, patients may intend to follow through with behaviors, but not all of their intentions are carried out; intentions can change with time. Unanticipated events and new information intervening between intention and behavior can influence intentions, attitudes, and subjective norms. In short, the TRA is a better predictor of attempts to do the behavior than of sustained performance of the behavior (Ajzen, 1988).

The theory of planned behavior (TPB) was developed in response to these limitations of the TRA. The TPB is based on the principles of the theory of reasoned action (Ajzen, 1991), but the TPB recognizes that attitudes and subjective norms are associated with attempts to perform behaviors. The strength of the attempt is a function of how much control the person has over personal and external factors that could interfere. For behaviors that require high levels of skill, the TPB suggests that the person develop an adequate plan to overcome these personal and external barriers. This suggests that problem-solving skills should be taught along with any new and complex health behavior. The TRA may provide an appropriate framework for the earlier example of the person with diabetes who has little difficulty with dietary recommendations at home, but the TPB may be more useful when the goal is ensuring the performance of dietary recommendations when that person is traveling or eating in restaurants. The TPB would suggest that intervention should include procedures to help the person develop contingency plans for maintaining proper diet under these difficult situations.

The theory of planned behavior also states that planning should include contingencies for failure of the behavior. Patient education based on the TPB that is focused on persons with diabetes would include strategies to identify personal and environmental factors that make it difficult to get the proper diet and would, with guidance (from the health educator), develop contingencies (e.g., arrange for a special meal on an airline flight, pack food for trips, inquire ahead about special meal options at restaurants, be the first to order in a restaurant). Clearly, the TPB has an advantage over the TRA in situations where the person has limited control over the behavior. Another advantage of the

TPB is that it focuses on the consequences of failure and the development of contingencies under personal and situational barriers leading to failure. However, both the TRA and the TPB are quiet about long-term behavior change and the event of a relapse in the behavior. Also, all models discussed to this point have little to say about persons who fail to participate even initially in patient education programs. The model discussed in the next section addresses some of these issues.

¤ TRANSTHEORETICAL MODEL OF BEHAVIOR CHANGE

One important aspect of behavior change involves understanding how an individual moves through the process of behavior change until the point where the behavior becomes a habit. One model that focuses on the transition points in the behavior change process and the underlying factors that facilitate transition from one stage to another is the transtheoretical model (TM). There are two major components to the TM that are relevant to the discussion here: stages of change and the process of change (Prochaska & DiClemente, 1983; Prochaska, DiClemente, & Norcross, 1992). In the *stages of change* component, it is assumed that persons move through discrete stages in the process of fully adopting the behavior. Individuals do not necessarily proceed in linear fashion; rather, they may cycle through stages of precontemplation, contemplation, preparation, action, and maintenance. *Precontemplation* is the stage at which there is no apparent intention to change behavior, at least in the foreseeable future. Persons in this stage include unmotivated individuals who may have unsuccessfully tried to change their behavior as well as persons who are truly unaware of the need to change their behavior. In either case, these individuals tend to be nonparticipants in patient education programs or nonrecruited patients.

Contemplation is the stage at which people are aware that a problem exists and are seriously thinking about changing their behavior. A key to defining this stage is that the person is seriously considering changing his or her behavior and is often very aware of the costs and benefits of the behavior change. However, at this point, the barriers and costs of behavior change are more compelling than the benefits. *Preparation* is the stage at which persons have taken small steps to engage in the behavior but have not yet taken effective action. Persons in this stage are assumed to be good candidates for patient education programs in that they are the most receptive of any in the three nonparticipant groups (precontemplation, contemplation, and preparation stages) about moving to the action stage. However, it should be noted that in some cases, a person may move very rapidly through these first three stages. For example, a person who has had a heart attack may readily take part in an exercise, weight loss, or smoking cessation program.

Action is the stage at which persons have begun to modify their behavior and are participating appropriately. Given the complexity of many patient education behaviors, the criteria for behavior compliance in this stage can vary considerably. For example, you may decide that persons in the action stage for hypertension medication adherence should be in total compliance, whereas persons in the action stage for exercise may be doing some exercise (say once a week for half an hour per exercise session) but have not yet reached the prescribed level (three times per week). *Maintenance* is the stage at which persons have begun to stabilize the behavior and it has become routine. The difference between the action and maintenance stages is similar to that between a behavior and a habit. Persons in the maintenance stage are less likely than those in the preceding stages to revert to their previous ways, are more confident that they will continue, and are likely to report that the behaviors are automatic and require little thought.

A relapse is considered to be movement from one stage back to the previous stage. The stages-of-change component also include a time reference to help identify stage transitions. For example, persons in the precontemplation stage for smoking cessation or who are adopting a routine of regular exercise include individuals who have no intention of adopting the behavior in the next 6 months. Similarly, the transition from the action to maintenance stage is typically defined as including those individuals who have performed the behavior for at least 6 months. The stages of precontemplation, contemplation, and preparation can be thought of as stages of readiness to adopt a behavior, whereas action and maintenance stages can be thought of as indicating the strength of the behavior once it is performed.

The *process of change* component of the TM states that specific processes and factors can facilitate the transition from one stage to the next. Much of the research (and theory development) identifying processes critical to the transition between stages has been focused on addictive behaviors and substance abuse and, more recently, on exercise, dietary behavior, and compliance with medication regimes. The model recognizes that stages can be stable and open to change and that these processes of change are common across behaviors. However, it is not likely that persons will proceed to action and maintenance stages unless the intervention matches the specific processes that facilitate the transition from one specific stage to the next. Some of the processes that have received the most attention include consciousness-raising, dramatic relief, self-reevaluation, environmental reevaluation, self-liberation, helping relationships, counterconditioning, contingency management, stimulus control, and social liberation.

Consciousness-raising is the process of increasing awareness and is important in the transition between precontemplation and contemplation. Any activities, such as reading information pamphlets and listening to physicians' recommendations, that can bring the person to awareness of the behavior are critical first steps in the transition to consideration of adopting the behavior. However, if the person is already aware of the need to change behaviors—for example, of the need to quit smoking—continuing to work on awareness will probably only alienate him or her. Dramatic relief includes any procedure that can help the person deal with the emotion associated with the behavior. This also facilitates the transition to a contemplation stage. For example, you might ask a smoker what he or she fears might happen if he or she stops smoking, or you may have the smoker meet with a former smoker who tells his or her own guilty story. Alcoholics Anonymous and other 12-step programs use dramatic relief to great benefit. Both self-reevaluation and environmental reevaluation include assessment of oneself and one's social interaction when performing or not performing the behavior. For example, you might ask a depressed patient to keep a daily exercise, mood, and energy diary to help him or her discover the connections among these three factors. Again, 12-step programs are excellent at helping participants evaluate their social and environmental interactions, and the frequency of meetings helps to build healthier social interactions. Reevaluation can be enhanced through a variety of methods, including mental imagery.

The transtheoretical model of behavior change is useful in patient education interventions for providing a framework for tailoring your program to the stage of readiness of the patient. It may not change what you do in the patient education program, but it may change when you do it. For example, you may have a component in your program that focuses on reinforcing appropriate behaviors in the context of self-care for arthritis. The TM would probably suggest that you focus on this type of strategy when facilitating the transition from action to maintenance, rather than at earlier stages. Of course, principles of behavior modification would suggest the same strategy. The value of tailoring the patient education program to the stage of the participant may also suggest cost-effectiveness over more comprehensive programs with no reference to staging. One way of accomplishing this is by avoiding prescribing behaviors; rather, allow the patients to choose which behaviors they want to work on at a given time. Although this may not accomplish all the behavior change you want, it usually does achieve some behavior change. Some is better than none.

Another potential benefit of the TM is that it provides a method for evaluating intermediate levels of patient success. It can be very frustrating to develop a patient education program in which the participants do not exhibit lasting behavior change. Using stages of change as a marker of success, you may discover that the program was very good for moving patients from one stage to another (e.g., contemplation to preparation) but not in reaching the final objective (the maintenance stage). Instead of starting over, an evaluation based on a stages-of-change framework may suggest a follow-up program to minimize program attrition and develop adherence, rather than program recruitment and initial participation. However, you first need to be careful with this approach. The association between stage change and maintenance is only weak to moderate. Second-stage change, although good for planning evaluation, is not an acceptable evidence-based outcome.

There are also potential problems that preclude the use of the TM in patient education programs and interventions. First, not all behaviors, especially complex behaviors and behaviors that need to be modified frequently based on disease activity, lend themselves to a stages-of-change analogy. A stage approach to patient education is unhelpful for complex behaviors that include an array of activities with no clear staging. For example, if the targeted goal is to provide the patient the necessary competence and skills to analyze and cope with unanticipated difficulties associated with management of heart disease, a stages-of-change theoretical approach would probably not be appropriate.

CEDE-PROCEED MODEL

λ..e precede-proceed model goes beyond stages of change, intentions, and perceptions (Greene & Kreuter, 1991). This model moves beyond the individual and the performance of specific health practices to include more of an ecological perspective on health education programs. It was developed mainly as a framework for planning and carrying out health promotion programs, but it has some applicability for patient education. This model looks not only at the individual perceptions and beliefs that influence behavior but at the larger social environmental influences, as well as the supports and resources, that reinforce the behaviors. Finally, the model focuses on the process of planning and evaluating health education programming.

There are eight stages in the precede-proceed model. The stages in the first part, or *precede,* take into account the influences that shape health status. The stages in the second part, or *proceed,* incorporate evaluation techniques and assist in policy development and implementation. The first step in the model involves making a social diagnosis about the target population (in this case, a patient population). *Social diagnosis* is defined as the process of determining people's perceptions of their own needs or quality of life and their aspirations for health and well-being. This is similar to the needs assessment discussed in Chapter 1. You may have decided on measures for quality of life for your patients, including getting back to work, self-management of medications, and independence of others for performing medical self-care. In order to assess people's perceptions properly, your program would need to involve members of the community to determine what they feel their needs are. An initial strategy you might use to accomplish this is to hold focus groups with your patient populations to determine their priorities and needs (see the discussion of focus groups in Chapter 1).

The second stage in the model is to identify specific health goals or problems that may contribute to the social goals or problems noted in the social diagnosis phase. Unlike the first stage, this step can be accomplished through inspection of existing literature and epidemiological evidence. For example, a major concern noted in the literature for persons with diabetes is foot care, and on the basis of your review of the literature, a major component of your program will include proper care for the feet.

The third stage involves identifying the health-related environmental and behavioral influences linked to the health problem you have found to be most deserving of attention through your work in the second stage. The behavioral part of this step recognizes that individuals play a major role in improving and maintaining their health. Your program should consider reviewing the findings related to the health risks. In the case of proper foot care, this may include the use of alcohol, inappropriate diet, and other related risk factors. This will give you an idea about which behaviors are most imperative to attend to within your program. A review of the literature is always very important; indeed, you may find that some of your own beliefs may not be well borne out in the literature. For example, the empirical evidence that stress reduction techniques can lower hypertension is weak. Environmental factors are also examined in this stage, including the social contexts and resources of the patients. In reviewing these factors, you might find that persons who live alone or who have few resources at home or in the community should also be incorporated into the program. It is possible, for example, that some patients do not have reasonable options in their immediate community for maintaining appropriate diet or do not have resource options for regular and safe exercise. It may be that part of your program will be directed toward the community to help provide the resources needed. As a result, you may decide to work with local food banks and soup kitchens to encourage them to supply appropriate foods for diabetics.

The fourth stage begins with the behavioral and environmental conditions identified as important in the third stage. The task in this stage is to identify the factors on which health education can have direct and immediate impacts on program results. These factors are categorized into predisposing, enabling, and reinforcing factors. Predisposing factors include the attitudes, beliefs, and values related to motivating the person to act. These might reflect a variety of the factors identified in the theoretical models previously discussed. For example, among diabetics, perceived lack of seriousness of problems pertaining to their feet, concerns with their ability to monitor and care for foot problems properly, and beliefs that an inappropriate diet has little impact on the course of their health may contribute to participants' lack of responsible foot care. This is also the place for media campaigns that might focus on the need for accessible public transportation for those with disabilities.

The fifth stage of the model marks the start of actual program implementation. This stage requires that you review what resources are needed and available to your organization by conducting an inventory of the resources available and those still required to implement a successful program. Then you are ready to select the appropriate combination of elements for your program's success. For example, on the basis of a review of resources available, you come to the realization that you have limited resources to affect the community. Based on this, you may decide to incorporate family members into your diabetes program to help them organize the community to support the resource needs of persons with diabetes, or you may decide that you can reach more people with Internet virtual discussion groups than with traditional face-to-face groups.

After all of the components are in place, the program can begin. The first five stages of the model provide the opportunity for the program organizer to review systematically the various factors that affect health and the resources that can be employed to address the health risk. This leads to the sixth stage of the model—the implementation phase. It also marks the transition from *precede* to *proceed.*

The seventh, eighth, and ninth stages of the model all involve evaluation. The seventh stage is the process evaluation phase, which focuses on whether the components of the program have been implemented as designed and whether the patients have been sufficiently exposed to program activities as well as on participants' reactions to the program activities and materials. (Process evaluation is discussed further in Chapter 3.)

The eighth stage involves impact evaluation and focuses on measurement of the effects of the program on a given set of behaviors. The final stage involves outcome evaluation. This type of evaluation returns the program to the earliest stages of development and examines those levels of health status and quality of life that were determined to be important in the first two stages. Has health improved? Has the quality of life in the community and of group members in the community gotten better?

Although the precede-proceed model is an excellent one for use in planning an intervention from needs assessment to evaluation, its focus is more on community interventions than on interventions for patients. In addition, the model has been developed mainly for health promotion rather than patient education. Finally, the precede-proceed model does not provide as much detail for planning the process components of intervention as do some of the theories and models discussed above. Nevertheless, it can be a very useful tool for those who must plan patient education interventions.

¤ A WORD ABOUT MONITORING AND SOCIAL SUPPORT

We have addressed the topic of monitoring only briefly in this chapter, and it deserves further attention. Patients are often surprised when they realize how much they eat, what they eat, how little exercise they get, or how much alcohol they drink when they start keeping track of these activities. Personal diaries of these behaviors provide a real sense of what people do for their health, whether they are at risk for health problems, and how far they are from recommended levels of behavior. You may wish to include monitoring procedures such as personal health diaries as part of your program. These not only serve as a useful method to help patients become aware of their behaviors; they also provide records over time that can help participants monitor their own success. Monitoring can also be used to help ensure that patients are adequately observing the appropriate outcomes of your program.

A related concept is the use of personal indicators and outcome measures of success. Regardless of your specific outcome measures of success, your program participants may have their own preferences and priorities in terms of outcomes. Having patients chart their own progress using their own meaningful indicators that are sensitive to your intervention is a good way to keep their motivation high. For example, if your program includes an aerobic exercise component and participants express concern over their inability to climb stairs, you could ask them to monitor how many stairs they can climb before they are tired and need to rest.

The use of social support is frequently incorporated into patient education programs. Social support is more then just encouraging and motivating people during the patient education program. It is supporting the person's commitment to being in the program and, often, to making lifestyle changes. There are many ways to encourage social support. You may ask patients to let their friends and family members know that they have joined the program. This should also be accompanied by specific efforts in your program to gain the support of family and friends for the patients (see the discussion of the theory of reasoned action, above). Another strategy for promoting social support is to encourage each participant to select a buddy in the program. Many patients will have brought friends with them or will be willing to make new friends through a buddy system. Patients can carpool to class, call their buddies to remind them about class, and support each other during difficult times in the program; all such social supports may help ensure adherence to the patient education program.

Although we usually think of social support as receiving support, we also need to consider the value of giving support. When our colleagues and we ask patients what they found most meaningful about the programs in which they participated, they often answer, "Sharing." When we ask them what they mean by that, they tell us that the programs gave them an opportunity to help others. On the surface, this may seem like a strange response. However, when people are ill, they often lose the helper role that many of us find important. If your patient education program is structured in such a way as to enable people to give support as well as receive it, the program may be all the more powerful. This was recognized many years ago by Irv Yalom (1975) when he identified altruism as an important therapeutic tool.

✪ SUMMARY

To use theory in creating a patient education program, you must first be very clear about what you are trying to accomplish and then must decide what content you are going to teach and how you are going to teach it (process). A general rule is to restrict the content to key messages. As we know, knowledge alone does not bring about behavior change. Try to keep your key messages to three or four per hour of teaching.

Next, choose the theory or theories that you are going to use to create your process. It is not enough to say that you want to empower people, so you will use self-efficacy theory. If you choose this theory, then you must systematically implement processes that include skills mastery, modeling, interpretation of symptoms, and other physiological states and persuasion. Here is another rule of thumb: If lectures, question-and-answer sessions, or both take up more than about a third of your education time, you are probably not using theory as effectively as you might. Just as it is difficult to change health behaviors, it is difficult to change educational behaviors. We all tend to do what is comfortable. If you have never systematically used theory, start by making small changes, arrange to observe a theory-driven program, talk to colleagues, or use the Internet to gain social support. Sound familiar? It should. This summary is aimed at persuading you to create theory-driven interventions. The decision to do so is up to you.

◘ BIBLIOGRAPHY

Ajzen, I. (1988). *Attitudes, personality, and behavior.* Chicago: Dorsey.
Ajzen, I. (1991). The theory of planned behavior. *Organizational Behavior and Human Decision Processes, 50,* 179-211.
Ajzen, I., & Fishbein, M. (1980). *Understanding attitudes and predicting social behavior.* Englewood Cliffs, NJ: Prentice Hall.
Bandura, A. (1997). *Self-efficacy: The exercise of control.* New York: W. H. Freeman.
Bandura, A., & Strunk, D. (1981). Cultivating competence, self-efficacy, and intrinsic interest through proximal self-motivations. *Journal of Personality and Social Psychology, 41,* 586-598.
Becker, M. (1974). The health belief model and personal health behavior. *Health Education Monographs, 2,* 324-473.
Borg, G. (1982). Psychophysical bases of perceived exertion. *Medicine and Science in Sports and Exercise, 14,* 377-381.
Clark, N., & Dodge, J. (1999). Exploring self-efficacy as a predictor of disease management. *Health Education and Behavior, 26,* 72-89.

Eng, E. (1993). The Save Our Sisters Project: A social network strategy for reaching rural black women. *Cancer Supplement, 72,* 1071-1077.

Fries, J. F., & Crapo, L. M. (1981). *Vitality and aging.* San Francisco: W. H. Freeman.

Greene, L. W., & Kreuter, M. W. (1991). *Health promotion and planning: An educational and environmental approach.* Mountain View, CA: Mayfield.

Janz, N., & Becker, M. (1984). The health belief model: A decade later. *Health Education Quarterly, 11,* 1-47.

Kaplan, G. (1997). Behavioral, social and socioenvironmental factors adding years to life and life to years. In T. Hickey, M. A. Speers, & T. R. Prohaska (Eds.), *Public health and aging* (pp. 37-53). Baltimore, MD: Johns Hopkins University Press.

McElroy, K., & Crump, C. (1994). Health promotion and disease prevention: A historical perspective. *Generations, 18,* 9-17.

McGinnis, J., & Foege, W. (1993). Actual causes of death in the United States. *Journal of the American Medical Association, 270,* 2207-2212.

Prochaska, J., & DiClemente, C. (1983). Stages and processes of self-change in smoking: Toward an integrative model of change. *Journal of Consulting and Clinical Psychology, 5,* 390-395.

Prochaska, J., DiClemente, C., & Norcross, J. (1992). In search of how people change: Application to addictive behaviors. *American Psychologist, 47,* 1102-1114.

Yalom, I. (1975). *The theory and practice of group psychotherapy.* New York: Basic Books.

3

Do I Know Where to Go, and Will I Know When I Get There?
Evaluation

Kate Lorig

When you have completed the first steps of developing a patient education program, needs assessment and choosing a theoretical base, the next step is planning your evaluation. In planning a good program, you must consider evaluation early. It is an important step in clarifying program goals. All too often, evaluation is an afterthought, not an integral part of program planning. This chapter examines the questions to ask, types of evaluations, and evaluation design. By considering evaluation early, you can avoid problems and shape your program toward the outcomes you are trying to achieve. Let us look at some examples of evaluation as an afterthought:

- I wonder whether our stop-smoking program was successful. We know that 1 year after the program, we had a 30% quit rate. However, we do not have a control or comparison group (we just did not think about it soon enough). Therefore, we do not know if 30% is good or bad. (In fact, this is a 1-year quit rate that is average or better.)
- I sure would like to ask the mothers who came to our children's health fair what they found most useful. Unfortunately, I do not have any way of contacting them. In fact, I do not even know who came–just how many.
- I wonder if people who were referred to our weight-loss program by doctors lost more weight than those who answered advertisements in the newspaper. However, I do not know how people learned about the program.
- People who took our diabetes course seem to be hospitalized less. I wish I had data to prove this. Our hospital administrator would be impressed by a cost-effective program.

Before discussing evaluations further, let us discuss some of the basic vocabulary and concepts. Please do not skip this section. By being able to speak the same language and truly understand the concepts, you will not be thrown off base when someone challenges your evaluation as "subjective" and therefore "not valid."

¤ SOME EVALUATION WORDS

Many special terms are used to describe evaluations. These allow communication but are also sometimes used as a secret language or as a means of intimidation. The important thing to know is that there is no one right way to conduct evaluation. Rather, good evaluations are part art and part science. Even the very best evaluators are learning new things every day. The following are some common evaluation terms. Being familiar and comfortable with them should serve you well.

Process or Formative Evaluations

Process or formative evaluations ask questions about how your program is operating. In other words, you are evaluating the process. These evaluations can be very simple or quite complex. Process questions include the following: How many people attended? Where did people find out about the program? Were some classes better attended than others? What was the dropout rate? Were the people who dropped out like the people who stayed, or were they different? How did the people who participated differ from the general population? Process evaluations can also be used to find out whether the program is being implemented according to a set protocol and whether the teachers are liked by the participants.

Outcome or Summative Evaluations

Outcome or summative evaluations ask whether your program is doing what you wanted it to do. Most commonly, outcome evaluations ask questions about changes in behaviors, health status, or health care utilization. However, sometimes you may put on a program with the express purpose of improving patient satisfaction. If this is the *purpose* of your program, then satisfaction could be an outcome, although it is usually a measure of process. The key consideration is the *intended outcome* of your program and whether you are evaluating this. Of course, if you are not clear about what you want a program to do, it is very hard to evaluate outcome.

Quantitative Evaluation

Quantitative evaluation collects data that are easily converted into numbers. It can be used for either a process or an outcome evaluation. Examples of quantitative evaluations are as follows:

- Asking participants to rate instructors on set scales
- Using instruments to measure depression, satisfaction, disability, and so on
- Using clinical data such as blood pressure or blood glucose
- Using chart or self-report data on utilization, such as the number of nights in hospital or the number of emergency-room visits

Quantitative evaluations are best used when you are very clear about the question that you want answered—that is, when you have a hypothesis. If you have a clear hypothesis, then almost anything can be quantified.

Qualitative Evaluation

Qualitative evaluation collects data that are not easily converted into numbers. (Even qualitative data can often be converted to numbers, but this takes thought and skill.) Qualitative data are almost always words. They are collected by means of semistructured interviews, focus groups, listening to the conversation of others, open-ended questions, collecting messages from Internet discussion groups, and through observation.

Qualitative evaluations are best when you are not at all clear about what is happening or when you do not know exactly what question to ask. These evaluations are often used to form a question or a hypothesis for a quantitative study.

To make things even more complicated, both quantitative and qualitative methods can be used in the same evaluation. For example, you might ask a series of questions about depression, health status, and behaviors, and then ask an open-ended question about what participants found most useful from an intervention.

A note of caution: All too often, I have heard patient educators say that they can't evaluate something or that more importance should be placed on qualitative data. First, anything can be evaluated. It is just that some things are harder to evaluate than others. I agree that more importance should be given to "good" qualitative studies. Unfortunately, most qualitative studies are poorly done. It is my experience that solid qualitative evaluations are much more difficult and time-consuming than are quantitative evaluations.

Objective and Subjective

Objective and *subjective* are words that are often used to confuse or intimidate the beginning evaluator. In theory, *objective* refers to anything that can be verified by a standard test and outside observation. Such data as blood pressure, cholesterol levels, and number of visits to a doctor are considered objective. *Subjective* refers to any data that can be biased by or that are the opinion of the reporter. Subjective data are considered not to be valid or "real" and are therefore suspect.

The problem is that the line between objective and subjective is not at all clear. Let us examine self-reports of visits to physicians (considered by some to be subjective) as contrasted with chart audits (considered by some to be objective). It is true that an individual may over- or underreport the number of visits or may confuse a visit to a lab with a visit to a doctor. However, a chart audit may also have problems. The individual may see several doctors at different places, and not all the charts may be audited, leading to underreporting of visits. The person doing the chart audit may count as only one visit seeing a primary care physician and then being referred to a specialist on the same day. At the same time, the automated record system may record allergy shots given by a nurse in an allergy clinic as a visit to a physician. Thus chart audits are not always valid.

Other examples of objective data are blood pressure and cholesterol level. Many people have been declared hypertensive on the basis of blood pressure readings taken in a physician's office. In fact, their blood pressure may be high because of anxiety surrounding a visit to the doctor. As for cholesterol level, laboratory data sent to five different labs have a good chance of getting several different cholesterol readings, some as much as 20 to 30 points apart.

The point is that seemingly objective data can be subject to bias. At the same time, subjective data can be valid. For example, pain and stress are always subjective. The important issue is not objective versus subjective but rather whether the data are valid. Do not ever let anyone intimidate you by questioning the objectivity of your data. Be prepared to explain why you believe that the data are *valid*.

Valid

Valid is the key word in the collection of any type of data. For data to be valid, they must meet two tests. First, you must get the same answers if you do the same test or ask the same questions twice within a short period of time. This is called *reliability*. However, something can be reliable without being true. For example, take a clock that is 15 minutes fast; five people look at the clock and report the same time. The data are reliable, but they are not correct. For something to be valid, it must be both reliable and correct.

To determine the correctness or validity of data, we usually compare it with some gold standard. For example, we have an

individual self-report his or her disability and then have a physical therapist (PT) give the person a series of tests and report the
disability. If the two reports are the same, then the self-reported
data are usually considered valid because they are the same as
the gold standard or the rating of the PT.

◘ EVALUATING INSTRUCTORS
(A PROCESS EVALUATION)

Often we ask participants to evaluate a patient education
program. Unfortunately, many times these evaluations are not
very helpful. When we ask people what they like best about a
program, the answer is often "Everything," and when we ask
them what they do not like, they sometimes still say that they like
everything. Such evaluations leave us feeling that we have excellent programs when this might not be the case at all.

To get better information, you might ask the following three
questions:

1. If you could keep only three things in this program, what would
   you keep? (Please do not say "everything"; we really want to
   know what three things you found most useful.)

2. If you had to get rid of three things in this program, what would
   you take out? (Please be as specific as possible.)

3. What would you like added to this program? (Please think a
   minute and give us a specific idea.)

Instructors tend to receive very high evaluations unless they
are really terrible. In fact, they tend almost always to receive
scores of 3 or better on 5-point scales on which 1 is *poor* and 5 is
excellent. This leads you to think that all your instructors are good.
A better way of rating instructors is first to have a set of questions

that you use for all evaluations of all instructors. For example, one question might be "How well prepared was this instructor?"

Next, take all the answers you receive to this question for all your instructors over a 6-month period and find the average score and standard deviation (you can do this with most calculators or on your computer). Let us say that the mean (average) score is 3.8, with a standard deviation of .4. (If you remember your statistics, about two-thirds of your instructors will be within 1 standard deviation of the mean.) Now you know that any instructor with a score from 3.4 to 4.2 (1 standard deviation from the mean) is an average instructor. Those instructors with a mean rating of less than 3.4 (more than 1 standard deviation below the mean) are instructors whom you should watch; they clearly have problems. Those instructors with scores above 4.2 (1 standard deviation above the mean) are well above average and should be treasured.

One note of caution: When you use this method to evaluate instructors, you will always have some instructors who are more than 1 standard deviation below the mean. They may still be good instructors. You have to make this judgment. What this method tells you is that of all the instructors you have, they are the poorest.

One last point about getting participants' evaluations. It should be clear to participants that the instructor will not see the comments unless the participants wish it. We always offer participants envelopes in which they can seal their completed evaluation forms before handing them in.

◻ ASKING THE RIGHT QUESTIONS

The most important part of any evaluation is asking the right questions. All evaluations start with the same two questions: (a) What do you want to know? and (b) Who cares? or, put more nicely, What difference does it make? It is important to spend a great deal of thought and time answering these two questions. As soon as you start to do an evaluation, you will think of a million things that you would like to know. Then, just to complicate matters, all your colleagues will think of extra things that they would like to add to your evaluation. The result can soon become a 3-hour interview or a 50-page questionnaire. Stop! Decide on three to five things that are the goals of your program and that you most want to know. Stick with these. There are several problems with collecting a lot of data. First, the longer the evaluation, the fewer the people who will complete it. Second, when you are finished, you are likely to be swimming in data, and you will not have enough time to analyze everything you have collected. In short, use the KIS principle: Keep it simple.

The following patient education outcomes provide a general framework for deciding what you want to ask:

1. *Knowledge:* Did the participants learn what you wanted them to learn? (Note that knowledge gain is no longer considered an important patient education outcome and, if used, should be used only in conjunction with other outcomes.)

2. *Behaviors:* These are such things as exercise, medication compliance, communicating with physicians, and using an inhaler properly. Behavior measures answer the question, Are participants doing what you want them to do?

3. *Attitudes/beliefs:* Have you changed patients' beliefs about the condition or their confidence (self-efficacy) in being able to do something about symptoms? Satisfaction with the health care system or with your intervention is also an attitude measure.

4. *Health status:* This is the real bottom line. Measures include blood pressure, disability, fatigue, shortness of breath, pain, role function, and blood glucose levels. A subset of health status measures would be psychological measures, such as depression, anxiety, and health distress.

5. *Health care utilization:* Sample measures include number and type of outpatient visits, hospitalizations, nights in hospital, use of medications, and emergency-room use.

Note that we ask about nights in hospital rather than days in hospital. This is because many people have day surgery or other treatments for which they spend a day in the hospital but do not stay overnight. Because what we want to know about is the length of hospitalizations, we always ask for the number of nights in the hospital.

We have also learned that many people confuse urgent-care visits, after-hours visits, and emergency-room visits. Thus when seeking information about emergency-room visits, we ask about visits to hospital emergency rooms.

Once you have more or less decided on the questions you want to ask, put them to the acid test. Ask yourself, "Who cares?" If you cannot give a clear, concise answer without beating around the bush, you probably do not have very good questions. By the way, when your colleagues come up with extra questions, you can use the same test. Ask them, "Who cares?" As a rule of thumb, if an interview or questionnaire takes more than 15 minutes to complete, it is probably too long. (Please note, this is not true if you are doing research as opposed to program evaluation.)

✿ METHODS: HOW DO I FIND OUT WHAT I WANT TO FIND OUT?

There are two basic types of evaluation methods: qualitative and quantitative. Some people might label these as subjective and objective evaluations. Do not get caught in this trap! If these words still confuse you, reread the discussion earlier in this chapter of the terms *objective* and *subjective*. There is nothing inherently subjective or objective about either method, nor is one method better than the other. Rather, the best evaluations use both methods. The question, not the bias of the evaluator, should be the basis for your choice of evaluation method.

Qualitative Evaluations

Qualitative methods are often used for answering "messy" questions. Sometimes, we want to know why something happened—for example, why heart disease patients stopped smoking. One way of getting the answer is to make a list of all possible reasons and have the ex-smokers check off the answers. The problem here is that no one can make an all-inclusive list. You will get answers only to the items on your list, and you may miss the real reasons people stopped smoking. In this case, it would probably be better to use qualitative methodology. Just ask people why they stopped smoking. Then have three judges read all the answers and form a list of general categories. Compare the three lists of categories and form one list of categories. You should have no more than 10 to 12 categories in all. Now go back through all the answers and have each of the three judges fit every answer into a category. Finally, compare the category placements of the three judges. Hold a discussion among the judges until consensus is reached for any differences in opinion. If some responses do not fit into existing categories, form new categories. It is important that each response fit into a category (an "other" category does not count). Also, it is important that consensus be reached when there is a disagreement.

Now, you may think that this would be much easier if only one person did all the above steps. It is true that you would avoid disagreement, but you also might miss some of the most important material. For example, in a study of the problems of handicapped children in school, the children often mentioned problems with physical education courses. Two of the judges put these responses into a category of physical problems. However, the third judge, who had been a handicapped child, put these responses into the social problems category. She ultimately convinced the other judges to agree with her. As you can see, the solution to that problem is very different depending on whether you consider it a physical or social problem.

If the question is really important, you can take the themes generated by a qualitative study and use an incomplete block design questionnaire (see Chapter 1) to survey your population. This methodology combines the strengths of qualitative and quantitative methods to gather data about messy questions.

Generally, qualitative evaluations take more time than quantitative ones. However, they often result in perspectives that would have been lost if only quantitative data had been collected. Incomplete perspectives can lead to weak programs. For example, one evaluator doing a study of compliance asked cardiac patients how often they forgot to take their medications. She concluded that patients forgot 20%-40% of the time, so she built a program based on memory aids. Another evaluator asked cardiac patients why they did not always take medications as directed and found that medications were missed in social situations. They were also missed because of misinterpretation of symptoms; the patient felt better and therefore decided there was no need for the medication, felt worse and decided the medication was not helping, or suffered side effects and decided not to take the medication. Using these findings, the second evaluator based her program on rehearsal of medication taking in social situations and reinterpretation of symptoms. The second program is likely to gain greater compliance than the first.

In choosing between quantitative and qualitative evaluations, a good rule to follow is that if you are not sure what you need to know, use qualitative methods. Ask the people who know, usually the patients.

Very often when conducting evaluations, you ask questions of the wrong people or maybe not of enough categories of people. For example, sometimes you want to know why people drop out of classes or have very sporadic attendance. To find the answers, you often ask the instructors. Now, everyone has legitimate reasons for not coming to class occasionally—an aunt is visiting, the person went on vacation, a child was sick. But unless people are very angry, they will never tell the instructor that they were bored, the room was uncomfortable, or their classmates had bad body odor. Thus, if you want to find out why people dropped out, call them and ask. A few carefully worded, tactful questions over the phone can get you a large amount of information. (By the way, the instructor or anyone else the participants know should never be the one making these calls.)

One last point about asking qualitative questions. Experiment a little with wording. Remember that people generally do not like to be negative. Therefore, asking what participants did not like about the program will not elicit much information. Rather, ask what they would change in the program. Also, if you ask what people liked, the answer is often "Everything." Again, this is not a very helpful answer. Instead, ask, "If you could attend only two or three parts of this program, what would you choose to attend?" or "If you could keep only three parts of the program, what would you keep?" This type of question forces participants to make a choice without being obnoxious. If you do not know how to ask a question, ask it three or four different ways and see which way yields the most useful (note I did not say "the most favorable") answers.

Quantitative Evaluations

Most evaluators favor quantitative evaluations or those that collect numbers. These are generally easier to conduct, and somehow numbers seem more solid than opinions. In some cases this is true, and in others, it is not. You would not ask someone to give you his or her opinion about his or her blood pressure reading; you would take his or her blood pressure. On the other hand, as we have already seen, valuable data are often lost in quantitative evaluations.

Usually, quantitative evaluations are conducted using a questionnaire, clinical data, or data that have already been collected for something else. Let us look at the latter first. Suppose that you want to conduct a hypertension program and want to know how many hypertensive patients there are in your institution. You might take the blood pressure of everyone who walks in the door for a week. This would give you some idea. An easier approach would be to go to the pharmacy and find out how many prescriptions are given out for hypertensive medications during the week. Both of these data collection methods have many flaws. Today, with increasingly sophisticated medical information systems, you might be able to get the computer to generate the number of patients seen for a specific problem. Be careful to find out the number of people, not the number of visits.

✪ FINDING AND CHOOSING THE RIGHT QUESTIONS

In most quantitative evaluations, you need to ask one or more questions. The more questions you ask, the more burden you put on the responder (sometimes called *response burden*). In addition, the more questions you ask, the more data you have to clean, code, enter into a computer, and analyze. All this takes time. Therefore you are usually better off asking a few important, well-aimed questions than shotgunning and hoping you will hit something. It is very important to ask the "right" questions. In the following paragraphs, we examine how to locate and make decisions about which questions to ask. First, however, you should note Rule 1: *If at all possible, do not create your own questions!* Writing evaluation questions is an art and a science. It is usually done by people called psychometricians. Although this is a very useful skill and can certainly be learned, it is probably more than the busy practitioner wants to tackle.

So, if you are not going to write your own questions, how do you start? First, you must be very clear about what you want to know. This was discussed earlier, but let me suggest some more examples. Say you want to know whether someone is more empowered after an educational program. You must define *empowerment*. The literature contains many empowerment-related psychological constructs, such as coping, learned helplessness, locus of control, health locus of control, readiness to change, and self-efficacy. Each has a different definition, and in fact, each is different from the others. If you know only that you want to investigate "empowerment," you are rather like the forest ranger who reports that she wants to count "animals"; when questioned, she reveals she is not interested in fish or insects, just four-legged animals, and upon more questioning, she realizes that what she really wants to know is how many white-tailed deer there are living in a certain geographic area. You must be equally specific in deciding what you want to measure.

If you have only a general idea, go to the library and do some reading to help you narrow down your ideas. Talk with colleagues. The most important thing is to choose something you really want to know and define it clearly. This is called the *operational definition*.

Let us say you decide on self-efficacy but have no idea about how to measure it. You know from your previous work that self-efficacy is behavior specific. Therefore, if you are evaluating an exercise program, you want questions about exercise self-efficacy.

To find an exercise self-efficacy *scale* (a group of related questions), conduct a search of MEDLINE and PsycINFO using the keywords *exercise* and *self-efficacy*. You can find MEDLINE on the Web at http://www.ncbi.nlm.nih.gov/pubmed. If the resulting list is too long, narrow the search by adding the word *scale* or *instrument.* Look at the titles and abstracts to see whether any of the articles describe an exercise self-efficacy scale. If not, see whether there are one or two authors who have done several exercise self-efficacy studies. If so, call or e-mail and ask what scales they use. Another thing you can do is to read some of the exercise self-efficacy studies. The instruments used for data collection are almost always described or referenced.

So you have done all of the above and now have not only one scale but four. How do you make a decision? Can you take the best questions from each?

Before answering these questions, we must again define some terms. A *question* is just that, one question. Sometimes, one question will do; for example, "Check one: male _____ female _____." We would not, on the other hand, try to decide whether someone could cope by asking the question, "Can you cope?" For many outcomes, to get really good answers, we need a series of different but related questions. This series of questions is called a *scale* or an *instrument.* Sometimes, when we think we need only one question, using a scale may be more helpful. For example, in doing a study in a gay, bisexual, or transsexual community, we might ask questions such as the following:

1. What was your gender at birth? male _____ female _____

2. How do you identify yourself now? male _____ female _____

3. Have your external sex organs been surgically altered? yes _____ no _____

Having defined *question, scale,* and *instrument,* let us go to Rule 2: *Do not pick and choose questions or make major changes in questions.* A scale must be used as a whole. The questions are like pieces of a jigsaw puzzle–they fit together. If a question or piece is missing, you get only part of the picture.

Of course, as with everything else, there are exceptions. For instance, some scales have subscales. A coping scale may use different questions to measure cognitive coping, passive coping, and physical coping. When put together, these three subscales form a coping scale. If you are interested only in cognitive coping, you can use the cognitive coping subscale and forget the rest of the questions. Sometimes, when you read about a scale, you will find that it is made up of four subscales (sometimes termed *factors*). A factor is the same as a subscale. All the questions in a subscale or a factor relate to each other better than they do to the questions in another subscale. This is what one learns from a *factor analysis*. It is okay to use a factor or subscale without using a whole scale.

As a general rule, you should not change the wording of questions. Sometimes, however, you have to use common sense. For example, an American disability scale asks about the ability to turn off a faucet. This makes no sense in Australia, where a faucet is called a *tap*. In changing things, however, you have to be very careful. This same scale, developed in the 1970s, asks about "dialing a telephone." Today, most people do not use a dial when they make phone calls. However, changing the wording to "using a telephone" defeats the purpose of the original question, which is to determine finger and wrist function. The question might have to be changed to "turning a doorknob" or "using a computer mouse."

Suppose you have found several scales and are not planning to change them. How do you choose which one to use? First, let us assume that all the scales have been tested for reliability and validity (see the subsection above headed "Valid"). If you cannot find information to confirm this, then you should drop the scale from consideration.

Next, you should look at usability. Is the scale usable by the evaluator? If you are working with 20 to 30 subjects, the coding of a visual analogue scale, which requires measurement with a ruler, is fairly easy. However, if you have hundreds or thousands

of subjects, visual analogue scaling will require extra time and resources. Can the data be entered into a computer by use of a
scanner? Of course, if the answer is yes, you must consider the
cost of a scanner, and then you must consider the ability of your
population to fill out scanner sheets correctly. Does the scoring
of the scale require complicated computer algorithms (decision
charts), and, if so, do you have someone who can create these? Is
the coding straightforward or complicated? In general, the best
advice is to keep it simple.

Probably more important is the user-friendliness of the instruments. Length is important. Generally, the more questions,
the more missing data you will have. If you have too few questions, however, you may sacrifice validity or the ability to regis-
ter change (*sensitivity*). Decisions should not be made on the basis
of length alone. In one case, we tested two scales measuring the
same thing. One scale had 6 questions, and the other scale had 20
questions. Our population much preferred the 20-question scale
because the response choices (*once a week, twice a week,* and so on)
were much more understandable than the response choices on
the shorter scale (*frequently, sometimes, seldom,* and so on).

Second, are the questions and the responses understandable
to the people using the scale? You test this by trying out the scales
on a few people and asking them whether there are any problems.

Third, are the questions too personal, or do they anger people in some way? Are the questions relevant to the people answering them? Asking Hispanics in New York about their use of
tortillas probably is not wise. However, asking about rice and
beans, foods common in the Southwest and in Mexican, Central
American, and Caribbean Hispanic communities, may be more
productive.

Finally, are the questions repetitive? Asking the same thing
many different ways may increase your validity. At the same
time, this may tire people or make them angry because they
think you are trying to trick them.

¤ TIPS ON DATA COLLECTION

Data are essential for both needs assessment and evaluation. The results of these endeavors are only as good as your data. Therefore, if your data are not representative of the group or if they are incomplete, your results can be badly flawed. For example, if you want to know about patient satisfaction and you hand out questionnaires in the waiting room, your sample is made up only of those who have sought care. You are missing all the people who may be so dissatisfied that they have gone elsewhere. It would be better to mail questionnaires or interview all patients (or a random sample of all patients) who were seen during a specified time period. Choosing a representative sample is not always easy, but it is necessary if you are to draw valid conclusions.

The biggest problem is often getting complete questionnaires. Sending out a questionnaire once is not enough. In our patient education studies, we mail our questionnaires with a friendly letter. Within 2 weeks, we usually get back about 50%. Then we send a postcard reminder, followed in about 10 days by a telephone call. Finally, 4 to 5 weeks after sending the initial questionnaire, we send a second questionnaire. This process usually results in an 80%-90% return rate.

Getting the questionnaires back, however, is only the halfway point in collecting good data. The other half involves getting complete data. Returned questionnaires are of little use if important parts of the questionnaire are not filled in correctly or are blank.

There are several ways to avoid this problem. First, formatting of the questionnaire is very important. The following are some suggestions:

1. Put questions on only one side of each page. If you must use both sides, be sure to cue your subjects to turn each page over. If your questionnaire is in booklet form, you can more easily use both sides of each page.

2. When you have many lines of questions, shade every second or third line so that the people completing the questionnaire will not check off the wrong answers.

3. Do not try to shorten your questionnaire by using small type or compressing the questions. It is best to use 12- or 14-point type.

4. Put your questionnaires on colored paper (tan, yellow, pink) so that they are easy to find on a desk full of white papers. Use the same color for the whole evaluation.

5. Think of your coding before you print your questionnaire, and leave space and lines for coding on the right side of the questionnaire. This is very important for computerized data entry. The entry persons should have to read only down the side of the page, not search out each answer. This process will also help you decide how to code answers and will help clarify what you really want to know and how to ask it.

Good questionnaire construction will save you many of the problems that can be caused by missing data or data that are impossible to interpret.

Having said all this, no matter how well you construct your questionnaires, people will find a way to mess them up. This puts you in the position of having to recapture data. If a whole page is missing, send the questionnaire back to the person with a nice note asking him or her to complete the missing page. Be sure to keep a photocopy of the questionnaire, so you do not lose any data already in hand.

If you just have a few questions that need clarification, send the person a postcard asking him or her to call you during office hours. Keep the questionnaires near the phone in alphabetical order so that questionnaires can be found easily. You can save much time by having people call you. Of course, you must be sure that the phone is answered by someone trained to collect the missing data.

If after a week a person you have contacted has not called, call him or her. Remember, many people work during the day, so you may have to call in the early evening.

When you are collecting data from the same person more than once, you will need to find him or her a second time. To help with this, on your first questionnaire, ask for the name, address, and telephone number of someone who will always know where the person is living. Then if the person becomes ill, moves, or dies, you will have another point of contact to pursue when you are doing follow-up.

Some populations are harder to get data from than others. This is especially true for follow-up data. Here are a few ideas from practitioner friends:

1. For a community survey of parents of young children, a short questionnaire was placed on the back of tray mats at a fast-food restaurant; the front side was left blank for artwork. Children were encouraged to draw pictures, and these were entered into a contest if the parents filled out the questionnaire on the back.

2. Women in jail were given a class on family planning and AIDS prevention. At the time of the class, they were asked for self-addressed envelopes to be used for follow-up questionnaires 6 months later. As an incentive for returning the questionnaire, each person was sent a state lottery ticket upon return of the questionnaire. A surprising 55% of the population was found and responded.

3. A needs assessment was conducted with medical residents. As an incentive for filling out the questionnaire, the names of those returning the questionnaire were entered into a lottery for dinner at a fine restaurant.

The information displayed in Table 3.1 may help you avoid some common questionnaire pitfalls.

TABLE 3.1 What Can Go Wrong With Questionnaires—and Usually Does!

Problem	Possible Reason	Possible Solution
They don't return the form.	Takes too much effort to get it back.	Make it easier. Send a stamped envelope. If local, make the return point as central as possible or pick up the forms yourself. Send a short, friendly letter explaining the study and offer an incentive.
They didn't even do them!	People have a right not to participate.	Remind them with a postcard or phone call.
	May not be as interested in the topic as you are.	Jazz it up. Try to increase their motivation to participate.
	Didn't understand what you wanted.	Call to get responses to a few important questions. Keep things as clear as possible. People don't struggle to understand; they're more likely just to throw the questionnaire away. Provide a sample response. Really good pretests would have shown a problem here.
They didn't answer all the items.	Not time enough?	Don't rush them. Call them. Don't ask too many questions for the time allowed or for the effort it takes.
They left an answer blank.	Maybe some were uncomfortable about answering, or the questionnaire was poorly formatted.	Try to eliminate unnecessary sensitive items. Try wording uncomfortable items carefully to minimize the reaction. May not be able to get at crucial stuff in the way; may need a relaxed, trusting interview. Place shading between every second question.
	Maybe they didn't know what to answer, had not enough information, or had no opinion.	Ask questions your sample would be expected to know.

continued

Table 3.1 Continued

Problem	Possible Reason	Possible Solution
	Maybe you didn't give them the choice they wanted.	At least at pretest, and if possible at test, leave one "Other (specify) _____."
They cut off my secret identifying code.	People aren't as dumb as they used to be.	Be open with your identification. Ask them to sign, but it has to be voluntary. (You risk getting fewer returned.) Don't bank on knowing exactly who they are.
On follow-up questionnaires, you cannot find participants.	They moved away or are deceased.	On the first questionnaire, ask them to provide the name, address, and phone number of someone who will know their whereabouts in 1 to 5 years.
They marked too many answers.	Maybe the choices you gave were not mutually exclusive.	If the choices are of the same kind, try to combine them into a single answer that reflects both parts.
	Questions and answers may have been spaced too close together.	Sometimes you can figure out which is the most likely to be the answer. Leave more space.
	Some answers depend on different circumstances.	Be prepared to jettison items or whole forms for those problems.
	Your directions were not clear.	Be sure initial directions are clear; repeat on each page. Indicate how many to mark. But some people just won't follow directions anyway!
They added their own answer.	Maybe you forgot a whole category of answers.	Hope you can include that on the next go-around. It is better to get this on the pretest, but you can't always be so lucky. Try to fit their answer within existing categories.
Everybody marked the same answer.	You picked a skewed sample.	Unless it's contraindicated, look for balance in other groups.
	You didn't break the answers down far enough.	Remove the item for reworking, retesting, etc.
	You asked an obvious question.	Dumb!
	You just confirmed a major trend.	Publish your finding fast.

continued

Table 3.1 Continued

Problem	Possible Reason	Possible Solution
I don't think they answered honestly.	May be hostile to tests, the situation, you, etc.	Try to win their cooperation. Be ready to toss out obvious goof-ups.
	May have a sense of humor, be drunk, etc.	Ditto.
	May be guarding confidential material.	If it is vital to know, use double items to check reliability. Be prepared to lose items. Try to figure out why they'd want to lie and judge what to do accordingly. The bottom line is, trust people; they usually tell the truth.
Why didn't I think to ask just that one other question?	Even researchers aren't omniscient.	Try a new form. Set up a dummy conclusion as completely as you can *before* you give the test; using your imagination this way can often suggest an omitted item. Try a new group with it added. Better luck next time.
They took so long to return it.	You didn't put a return date on it.	Place the date by which you need it where it's sure to be seen. Send a reminder a week or so after the due date to remind those who have not yet returned them. (This is where it pays to know just who has returned and who has not returned questionnaires.)

NOTE: Remember, always be nice; the participant is always right.

SOURCE: Archer, A., & Fleshman, R.: *Community Health Nursing.* © 1985. Boston: Jones and Bartlett Publishers. Adapted with permission.

Finally, you have all your data. Now what to do? Data analysis and statistics usually make the eyes of a patient educator glaze. Don't become catatonic. First, there are some good, easy-to-use statistics books for beginners (e.g., Brown & Beck, 1994; Kanji, 1993). You might be surprised at what you can do yourself. Even without a statistics book, you can do averages and tallies. This may be enough. For instance, you may be able to state results such as "A total of 30% of participants stopped smoking for 1 year," "Average class attendance was 4.2 out of 6 sessions," or "Participants lost an average of 5 pounds during the 10-week program."

Another useful tool for data analysis is Epi Info (see the final section of Chapter 1 for details). This inexpensive computer program is very user-friendly and comes with an excellent manual. The software is available for public access and thus can be freely shared.

Again, data analysis is a specialty for which you can get help. However, do not wait until the end of your project to talk with a statistician. The time to start talking is when you are beginning to think about evaluation. Statisticians are much more than number crunchers. If you get one interested in a project early, he or she can be a huge amount of help. Unfortunately, some statisticians do not speak English; they speak their own brand of professional jargon. If possible, avoid this type. By the way, you probably do not need a card-carrying statistician. Very often, someone with an advanced degree in one of the health sciences can help you.

✪ STUDY DESIGN

Like questionnaire design, study design is an art. There are several excellent books that will give you good ideas (see Green & Lewis, 1986; Windsor, Barabowski, Clark, & Cutter, 1994). The most important thing to remember is that quantitative evaluations need some type of comparison. Participants' condition after the program can be compared with their condition before the program. That is how we got the 30% quit rate for smokers. Sometimes, participants are compared several times. For example, you get exercise rates 4 months before the program, when the program starts, 4 months later, 8 months later, and 1 year later. This is a time series design and has the advantage of letting you know two things. First, did your program cause the change in exercise rates, or was the change caused just by time? You might find that 20% of the group started exercising in the 4 months before the program but that after the program, 70% of the group was exercising. This suggests that the program was responsible for getting 30%-50% of the group to exercise. By continuing to collect data, you can find out how long program effects last. If at 8 months only 10% of the population is exercising, then the program's effect didn't last very long. However, if at 1 year, 50% of the people are still exercising, you know that the program had a good long-term effect.

Usually, the strongest design is one that has a randomized comparison group. In this case, you would take all the people who were interested in a program and let half of them take the program while the other half are not allowed to take the program or are asked to wait for several months before taking the program. In this way, you can compare those taking the program with those not taking the program. When the two groups are randomly chosen, they are probably very similar. Therefore, any effects that you find are likely to be caused by your intervention and not by differences in the groups.

With a little bit of planning, you can have two evaluations for the cost of one and also use a randomized design. Let us say that you want to evaluate a new back pain class but that the PTs are very happy with the way that they are now giving one-on-one education. You might suggest that patients be randomly assigned to either the new group program or the old one-on-one program. All patients are evaluated before they start the program and again in 3 or 6 months. If one group of patients has better outcomes than the other group, then that method of giving education is clearly better. If both groups are the same, you have a dilemma. You know that both types of education are about the same, but you do not know whether they are both effective or are both ineffective. To answer this question, you would need a group that did not get a back pain program.

Most health education practitioners are reluctant to use a randomized design because they are afraid that those told that they cannot take the program will be angry. In reality, we have found that if people understand what you are doing and why, they are usually quite willing to wait a few months for their education. In 20 years at the Stanford Patient Education Research Center, we have had more than 5,000 people participate in randomized studies in which the controls have been asked to wait 4 to 8 months. We have seldom had any problems either getting or maintaining control groups.

If a randomized comparison group is not possible, then it may be possible to find a similar but nonrandomized comparison group. This could be made up of hypertension patients from another hospital. Or you might want to give your program in one part of the city and use people in another part of the city as controls. In any case, the important thing to remember is that the comparison group must be as similar to the treatment group as possible.

A word about evaluation and ethics. When it gets right down to conducting an evaluation, many practitioners are very concerned about the ethics of the study. They may feel that it is not ethical to deny people education, as might be necessary in a randomized design, or they may feel that people will be turned off when asked to answer questions. Sometimes confidentiality is an issue. In my experience, these concerns are most often voiced by health professionals and are seldom concerns of the lay public. If people are told why the evaluation is being conducted, are treated with respect, and are assured confidentiality, there are seldom objections.

It may be that before you can conduct an evaluation, especially if you are using a randomized design or are collecting data from patient records, you will have to get approval from your institutional human subjects committee or ethics committee. This is an extra hurdle, but it is often well worth the effort.

Even if you do not have to obtain signed informed consent, it is a good idea to include with your first questionnaire a letter worded in user-friendly English (or whatever language you are using) and states the purpose of the evaluation, who will see the data (only the study personnel—not participants' own health care providers, friends, or family), and how the data will be reported (only aggregate data—no data that will identify individuals). You should also give people a number to call if they have any questions.

Sometimes practitioners are threatened by evaluation or may not like it for other reasons. If such practitioners are the people who are collecting the data, they can sabotage your study. If the person presenting the study to patients displays a negative attitude about the study, then it is almost certain that you will have few participants and lots of missing data. On the other hand, if the person presenting the study is positive and excited about the study, you will get high participation rates and few missing data. In a recent study my colleagues and I conducted, we had more than 80% participation in groups that had positive presenters and approximately 25% participation in groups in which the presenters were negative. This means that it is vital to train those who first present the study and to ensure that all your presenters are positive.

The above discussion has been designed to give you a few ideas about the thought processes that go into any evaluation. You cannot become an evaluation expert overnight. Like anything else, evaluation is a skill. You need practice and guidance to become proficient. However, all practitioners can be good evaluators. Just do not be afraid to stick your toe into the water. You might even find that you like swimming!

¤ BIBLIOGRAPHY

Archer, A., & Fleshman, R. (Eds.). (1985). *Community health nursing: Patterns and practice.* Boston: Jones & Bartlett.

Brown, R. A., & Beck, J. S. (1994). *Medical statistics on personal computers.* Plymouth, England: BMJ.

DeVellis, R. F. (1991). *Scale development: Theory and applications.* Newbury Park, CA: Sage.

Green, L. W., & Lewis, F. M. (1986). *Measurement and evaluation in health education and health promotion.* Palo Alto, CA: Mayfield.

Kanji, G. K. (1993). *100 statistical tests.* Newbury Park, CA: Sage.

Windsor, R. A., Barabowski, T., Clark, N., & Cutter, G. (1994). *Evaluation of health promotion and education programs* (2nd ed.). Palo Alto, CA: Mayfield.

4

How Do I Get From a Needs Assessment to a Program?
Program Planning and Implementation

Kate Lorig
Margo Harris

Putting together a patient education program is a little like being a juggler: You have to keep several balls in the air at the same
time. The first ball is nearly always a needs assessment; the other
balls are launched more or less simultaneously. At the same time
that you are considering how to evaluate your program, you
should be launching the plan for its implementation. In other

words, you will have to make many decisions about what your program will look like.

¤ SETTING PRIORITIES: CHOOSING WHAT TO TEACH IN THE TIME ALLOTTED

Whether patient education is given in 5-, 10-, or 15-minute blocks or in several hour-long classes, you never have enough time to teach everything. Thus it is necessary to set priorities. In Chapter 1 we have addressed the usefulness of focus groups for determining key messages. The following three steps are also useful for helping you decide what to teach:

1. Listing all behaviors affecting the particular condition
2. Determining which behaviors are most important in affecting health status
3. Determining which behaviors are the easiest to change, given a limited amount of educational time

Note that all of these can be combined with the use of focus groups. Let us examine each of these steps in turn.

Listing Behaviors

For all health conditions, there are a number of behaviors that, if changed, would affect the condition. For example, someone with hypertension might be advised to stop smoking, lose weight, cut down on sodium, exercise, reduce stress, and comply with medication usage. A similar list can be made for any condition. The first step in setting priorities is to make a list of all behaviors that might affect the condition. In other words, you list everything you would like to teach.

Determining the Effect of Each Behavior

This is probably the most difficult part of priority setting. As health educators, we do not know a great deal about the relative effects of health behaviors on health outcomes. However, not all behaviors are equal. In lowering blood pressure, medication compliance and smoking cessation are probably the most important, with weight loss, sodium reduction, and exercise coming somewhere in the middle. Stress reduction, although very popular, probably has only a limited long-term effect on hypertension. Therefore, in choosing priority behaviors, you should first look at smoking cessation and medication compliance.

The question arises: How do you determine the relative effects? This is where you should use experts. Ask physicians or epidemiologists to help with this problem. You can also read the studies yourself. In recent years, the U.S. government has helped with these problems by sponsoring studies to determine the best practices for the treatment of various conditions. Most of these studies have been sponsored by the Agency for Healthcare Research and Quality (formerly the Agency for Health Services Policy and Research), and the resulting documents can be found on the Internet. For an index of AHRQ studies go on-line to http://www.ahcpr.gov/research. In addition, the Preventive Services Task Force has published an excellent book that outlines consensus recommendations for many conditions. This information can also be accessed on the Internet at http://www.ahcpr.gov/clinic/epc.

One important note of caution: Do not set priorities based on the popular press. For example, in recent years we have all been urged to cut down on dietary cholesterol. There is no question that blood cholesterol affects heart disease and that for someone with very high blood cholesterol, cutting down on dietary cholesterol may help. However, bringing about big changes in blood cholesterol usually requires medication. Most of the major studies that have found the lowering of cholesterol to reduce heart disease have accomplished the lowering of cholesterol primarily through medication usage. Our knowledge of the effects of lowering cholesterol through dietary means is much more fragmentary. This is especially true for the elderly. What does all this mean? Should we do nothing? No, we should continue to urge a low-cholesterol diet but also realize that this should not be at the cost of quality of life. The fad of today may well be seen as the mistake of tomorrow. Remember, 30 years ago we were urging everyone to eat red meat. In short, be responsible for knowing about the research base for behaviors that you are urging others to change. In addition, you should go back to your evaluation framework. If you are planning to evaluate changes in health status or changes in utilization, you will want to focus on behaviors that are most likely to have effects on these outcomes. If you are evaluating changes in behaviors, it is important that the behaviors reflect best practices and are consistent with what you teach. Next you will need to determine the ease with which behaviors can be changed.

Determining Which Behaviors Are Relatively Easy to Change

We all know that some behaviors are easier to change than others. For example, it is relatively easy to get someone to take a pill once a day and much more complex to get someone to bring and keep his or her weight down. The next step is to look at the items you listed as important to health and to rank how easy or difficult each is to change. One quick and not always accurate rule of thumb is that it is usually easier to get people to add behaviors than to give up behaviors. Depending on the amount of time, you can now choose which behaviors are most appropriate for your program. If you have only 10 minutes with a hypertensive patient, you might concentrate on medication compliance and lowering sodium intake. On the other hand, if you have 10 hours, you might work on diet, exercise, and smoking behaviors in addition to compliance and sodium reduction.

Another way of setting priorities is to let patients choose. Make a list of all the things that someone might do. For example, the list for losing weight might include not eating after 7:00 p.m., not eating between meals, broiling foods instead of frying them, cutting down on sweets, cutting down on fats, eating more fruit and vegetables, and increasing exercise. Then let patients choose the behaviors that they feel they can accomplish. This method has two advantages. First, you do not have to tell patients everything about dieting and exercise. If there is something on the list that they do not understand, they can ask. Second, patients are given choices and control. The more the new health behaviors are chosen rather than prescribed, the better the chance that they will be adopted.

In short, priority setting is based on the amount of time, the importance of the behavior, and the ease with which the behavior can be changed.

¤ REFINING YOUR CONTENT

Once you have decided on your target behaviors, the next step is to define what someone needs to know and what skills he or she must have to accomplish the behaviors. For example, patients with hypertension probably do not need to know the anatomy and physiology of the cardiovascular system. However, they do need to know the most effective ways to stop smoking and to remain nonsmokers. They need skills in fending off the social pressures to overeat and smoke, and they need to know how to change the environmental cues for smoking and eating. One of the greatest errors in many patient education programs is to spend a lot of time on interesting facts at the expense of learning and practicing necessary skills.

Sometimes refining content is almost self-evident. To comply with appropriate medication use, patients must know when to take the medication and how much to take. Often, to learn about necessary skills and knowledge, it is necessary to know the literature. In many areas of patient education, including smoking cessation, dietary changes, and exercise programs, there has been research on what patients need to know and do. You may have to juggle, but you don't have to re-create the whole circus.

A word of caution. All of the above may seem very sensible but not worth the time. Thus you may be tempted to do what you have usually done—that is, seek the opinions of various health professionals and then base your program on their input. Unfortunately, this will probably not lead to a strong program. Although you can certainly not leave out your professional colleagues, your patients deserve a program based on scientific knowledge and past studies rather than on individual beliefs and preferences. None of us wants to go to a physician who has not kept up with the changes in medical knowledge. In the same manner, patient education programs should be based on the latest information.

☒ SETTING OBJECTIVES

Once you have done your needs assessment and chosen your content, the next step is to write objectives. These objectives make clear what you are trying to accomplish and will serve as standards for evaluation. Just as there are two types of evaluations, there are two types of objectives: process objectives and outcome objectives.

Process objectives are those by which you determine the process of the patient education. Examples include the following:

- Fifty people will receive diabetes education this year.
- Publicity for the program will appear in six newsletters.
- Each participant will speak at least once at each session.
- Some 70% of the participants will make a contract for at least one behavior change.

Notice that in writing process objectives, nothing is said about changing health behaviors or health status. Instead, these objectives deal with managerial and teaching process.

Outcome objectives tell what we hope to accomplish in terms of changes in health behavior or health status. Examples include the following:

- After 2 hours of instruction, 70% of the diabetics will be able to self-inject insulin.
- By the end of the course, 80% of the participants will report that they exercise 120 minutes a week.
- After instruction, 60% of the patients will have a diastolic blood pressure below 90.
- Of the persons screened at the health fair and found to have high cholesterol readings, 60% will see a doctor within 1 month.

How to Write Objectives

All objectives have three parts: (a) an action, (b) criteria for the action, and (c) criteria for judging whether the action has been accomplished.

An Action

The action or verb part of the objective must be something that you can hear or see. Sometimes you can also use smelling or tasting verbs. However, these are not always useful in patient education objectives. *Report, eat, walk,* and *have a diastolic pressure* are good action words for an objective. On the other hand, *know, understand, think,* and *feel* are not good action words. There is no way that you can see someone knowing something. If your objective is that the participants will have more knowledge, then the objective should read, "Eighty percent of the participants will score 70 or above on a diabetes quiz" or "When asked to name their medications, 75% of the participants will be able to name all the prescription medication that they will be taking when they leave the hospital." "Participants will feel more in control of their asthma" is not a good objective. A better one is, "Eighty percent of the patients will increase their score by 10 or more points on an asthma self-efficacy scale."

Probably the most important part of writing an objective is choosing the correct action. The question to ask yourself is, Who cares? It is all fine and good that patients score well on a quiz. However, we know that changes in knowledge do not necessarily lead to changes in behavior or health status. If they did, we would have no smokers, alcoholics, overweight people, or people who do not floss their teeth. Thus knowledge objectives are probably not the best for most patient education programs. Instead, write objectives about what you want patients to accomplish by lowering cholesterol or blood pressure, stopping smoking, taking medications as directed, or following an exercise program. If the outcome does not make a difference, then it probably should not be included as an objective. Rereading the first part of this chapter on choosing content should help you in forming your objectives.

Criteria for the Action

This part of the objective answers the questions *who, what, when,* and *where:* for example, "after the course," "the participants," "the siblings of burn patients," "cholesterol or blood pressure reading," or "given a choice of cooking oils." If you do not know who is going to do something, and how, when, or where people are going to do it, then you have no way of judging whether or not it happens.

Criteria for Judging Whether the Action Happens

This part of the objective answers the question of *how many* or *how much*. It almost always deals with numbers: for example, "80% of the participants," "diastolic blood pressure of 90 or below," "increase at least 10 points," or "four blocks, three times a week." Without this criterion, you have no way of knowing whether you reached your objective. It is fine to say that patients will lower their blood pressure. However, you also need to know how many participants lower their blood pressure and by how much. Is a program successful if 2 of 100 patients accomplish what you want them to accomplish? Probably not.

You also have to know the starting point. If 70% of the people coming to a diabetes program are already able to read product labels, then an outcome objective that 80% will be able to do so at the end of the program does not represent meaningful change. On the other hand, don't be too optimistic. For example, it is not realistic to write an objective that 1 year after a smoking cessation program, 80% of those starting the program will not be smoking.

Objectives and Program Planning

Let us now look at how objectives can be applied to program planning. First, you should write only a few (fewer than 10) overall objectives for your program. These program objectives also form the basis for your outcome evaluation (see the subsection on outcome or summative evaluations in Chapter 3). Then write objectives for each session or patient encounter. For example, the overall objective for a hypertension course might be "At the end of the course, 70% of the participants will have a diastolic pressure below 90." The objectives for Session 1 of a hypertension course might be "Participants will (a) discuss three ways of lowering blood pressure and (b) choose one behavior they will change in the coming week."

In addition, process objectives should be written. These can usually be standardized for the entire intervention and do not need to be written for each session. For example:

> Instructors will (a) take attendance at every class, (b) ensure that all participants say something at every session, (c) reinforce verbally or nonverbally (with nods of head, etc.) every person in every class, (d) ensure that 80% of the participants make a commitment to some activity at the end of Sessions 2 through 6, and (e) use brainstorming as a problem-solving technique.

Such process objectives form the basis for your process evaluation (see the subsection on process or formative evaluations in Chapter 3). They also give your instructors a clear picture of what is expected and give you a means to evaluate your instructors. By simple observation, you can see whether the teachers are merely teaching content or are also using good patient education process.

In summary, objectives tell you where you are going and how you are going to get there. Writing them may seem burdensome. However, the very process of writing process and outcome objectives forces you to clarify your thinking. More important, writing objectives enables you to communicate what you are thinking to others. Finally, objectives give you standards by which to evaluate your program.

✪ PROCESS

By now you have chosen your content and written your objectives. The next step is to plan your process, or how you are going to teach. In achieving behavior change and changes in health status, process is at least as important as content and probably more important. As a general rule of thumb, it is a good idea to use several different processes each session. Also, the more interactive and participatory processes are, the more likely it is that change will occur. This section discusses a number of commonly used methods of patient education.

Media

Many people think of pamphlets, videotapes, or Web sites when they think of patient education. It is true that materials and media are very useful. However, seldom do they constitute a complete patient education program. Very few materials stand alone. Choosing and using materials is such a large topic that it is discussed here in its own chapter (Chapter 7).

Mass Media

Mass media can take many forms, each with its own advantages and disadvantages. For example, newspaper, radio, and television can reach large numbers of people and are excellent for making the public aware of a single need or event. It would not make much sense to use a small-group or even a lecture format to try to inform people about an impending flood. On the other hand, mass media messages are very expensive unless you use free public service announcements. The problem with free media is that you have no control over when your message will be released, or, sometimes, the exact content of the message. Getting good free use of the media requires a lot of press cultivation. Mass media messages, unless you can obtain a huge amount of media time and the message is very simple, are not good at changing health behaviors. Remember, stopping smoking is much more complicated than changing brands of detergent. On the other hand, mass media can be an important part of an integrated patient education program. For example, mass media can be used to give the public the message that people with back pain should continue to be active. This is an important message. This can then be backed with print material and with classes on how to remain active even when one is in pain.

Local Media

Local media are an often overlooked form of media. In most communities, local media provide some free public access. Although it is true that local media and newspapers sometimes do not have big audiences, they can be used in some creative ways. For example, the Stanford Heart Disease Prevention Project produced a group of smoking-cessation programs. The programs used a lecture/discussion format, and a local media personality went through the program on TV. People were urged to watch individually or in small groups. There was a great deal of advance publicity to let people know about the coming program. However, this was still a targeted audience of several thousand people. Of course, the production time and skills needed to use local media are fairly complex. Nevertheless, these can often be donated by students and others. In the United States, public-access cable stations offer free technical assistance. A final advantage of the use of local media is that if it is done skillfully, it can combine the advantages of mass media and small groups.

Computer-Based Education

Computers are now becoming widely available in schools, libraries, and homes. They represent a much-underutilized medium for health education. The advantage of computer-based education (CBE) is that it can reach large audiences. For example, there are CBE programs available on stress management, weight loss, and arthritis. These programs can be placed in schools and workplaces as well as in health care settings. With the advent of CD-ROM, people can also access the programs at home. Computer-based education can be somewhat individually tailored and can be paced to the needs of the individual. Once produced, it is relatively inexpensive. The disadvantage of CBE is that, as with any health education materials, good production requires both educational and technical skills. Also, CBE software must be compatible with the computers on which it will run.

Films and Videotapes

Films and videotapes are excellent if you know exactly why you are using any one in particular. Videos allow you to illustrate something, sometimes in a more entertaining way than you could in an ordinary educational setting. In addition, they can illustrate some skills that may be difficult to show in a class setting, such as exercise or food preparation. If patients have VCRs, they can take videotapes home to reinforce new behaviors. This is especially true for exercise programs. Videotapes may also be a means of providing education for patients with relatively rare diseases or with low reading skills. Finally, videotapes can be used to explain a new program to health professionals. For example, the Kaiser Permanente Health Care System has produced short videotapes that illustrate both group visits and the Living Well with Chronic Conditions workshops. These are shown to health professionals as the programs are being introduced throughout the United States. Sometimes a picture (or video) is worth a thousand words.

One last note: Audiotapes are much easier and less expensive to produce than videotapes. They can sometimes be an excellent substitute for videotapes.

The Internet

The Internet is an amazing health information and education resource, and it is right at your fingertips! Although they may not tell you spontaneously, many patients and/or their family members use this resource. Some use it extensively. The Internet can supply your patients with a wealth of information and resources, such as the following:

- The location and availability of clinical trials
- Access to the National Library of Medicine and medical journal citations
- Support groups for health conditions
- The latest health news
- Unlimited health information–from traditional to alternative

When it comes to use of the Internet, it is important that you establish a dialogue with your patients. Patients will ask you for reliable Internet resources, and you need to ask them what information they are accessing on the Internet. Ask them to share that information with you. Stress the point that a patient is an important member of the health care team and that all team members need to be well-informed. Encourage your patients to share information gained from the Internet or any other information source.

There are some basic tips and ideas you need to consider when you and your patients use the Internet. These include issues such as safety, credible information sources, currency of information and site addresses, and useful references. You may want to add more of your own ideas to this list.

Safety

Keep in mind this quote, which Ann Landers once used as her "Gem of the Day": "Be careful when you read health books. You could die of a misprint." Health information can be lifesaving, but it can also be potentially life threatening. The information on the Internet is also available from many other sources, including TV, books, radio, and magazines. But the information on the Internet is immediate. Some patients act on that information immediately–often without telling you.

Remind your patients and yourself that anyone can put anything on the Internet—and they do. Reassure your patients that accurate information is available on the Internet and that you want to work with them to help find that information and ensure its accuracy to keep them safe. Strongly encourage your patients not to change their health care plans based on information they find on the Internet without consulting you first.

Credible Information

Patients may think that because information is on the Internet, it is accurate and comes from a credible source. Encourage patients to identify the information source and learn more about that source before they accept the information shared on an Internet site. Remember that the site's domain name can give you and your patients insight into the source. An *.edu* extension in an Internet address identifies an educational organization. Other extensions are as follows:

.com = commercial
.org = organization
.gov = government
.mil = military
.net = network

Look for these address extensions and help patients understand that different site sponsors share different types of information. A commercial site (.com) that sells products may be more interested in selling you products than in providing you with accurate and objective health information. On the other hand, sites with an *.org* or *.gov* extension may offer more credible information and are good information starting points for patients and providers. Here are some examples of credible Web sites.

- Healthfinder, at http://www.healthfinder.gov/

- American Cancer Society, at http://www.cancer.org/
- American Heart Association, at http://www.americanheart.org/
- American Lung Association, at http://www.lungusa.org/
- Arthritis Foundation, at http://www.arthritis.org/
- National Institutes of Health, at http://www.nih.gov/
- PubMed (National Library of Medicine), at http://www.ncbi.
  nlm.nih.gov/pubmed/

If you are working with patients who have a specific health condition, you may want to compile a condition-specific list of credible health sites as starting points for patients interested in using the Internet. Gomez.com, which rates health sites, will help with this task. In addition, if the health condition is represented by a nonprofit organization, that site address could be included on your list.

Currency of Information and the Site Address

You and your patients want information that is up-to-date, and that is one reason to use the Internet. Be sure to check the dates on Internet sites. Most sites will include a reference to when the site was posted or when it was last revised or updated. The revision date may not apply to all pages on an Internet site, but it does give you an indication as to whether or not the site is being updated or reviewed.

Don't be discouraged if you type in an address for a Web site and discover that the address has changed. The Internet is dynamic, and site pages change every day. When a site address changes, just as with telephone numbers, you may be automatically forwarded to the new address. If you aren't forwarded, don't assume the site is gone for good. Choose one of the many Internet search engines available (e.g., HotBot, Yahoo, Metacrawler) and search for a new address by using the name of the organization or the old site.

There are several other ways in which you can use the Internet. You can create your own Web site and include all the information you usually give patients. One orthopedic surgeon we know has a wonderful Web page that includes easy-to-understand information about common surgeries along with photos and X rays. It also includes postsurgical instructions and exercises. Patients still meet with him and the physical therapist, but now they have a place to go if they "forget" or there is something they don't understand.

If you don't want to create a Web site, you might use e-mail to answer patient questions. Or you might create an e-mail list so that patients can communicate with you and with each other. In fact, you can have a virtual support group.

One last note: Most patients prefer e-mail lists to chat rooms. Lists are not dependent on real time. In addition, most chat rooms are very slow.

Useful References

When you think of useful references, consider people and print! Your local public library and local hospital or medical center library may offer help for you and your patients. It has been estimated that 70% of Internet searches are health related, and libraries work to respond to that interest. Librarians are great resources for locating print and electronic health information. An increasing number of public libraries have Internet access available to patrons. Local medical libraries may also offer information services to members of the community. If you know your library offers that type of service, share that information with your patients. Two good books for you to have on your own shelf and to share with patients are Ferguson and Madara's *Health Online* (1996) and Maxwell's *How to Find Health Information on the Internet* (1998).

Group Processes

Brainstorming

Brainstorming is one of the most common ways of gaining group participation in a nonthreatening manner. It is also useful for generating many ideas and for forming new ideas. Although it is often used, brainstorming is at times done incorrectly. Proper brainstorming consists of five steps:

1. *Give participants directions.* For example: "I will ask you a question, and then you should give as many ideas as you can. Do not worry if the ideas sound silly or are a little strange. If you do not understand what someone else says, do not worry; we will talk about this later. Right now, all I want is for you to give as many ideas as you can."

2. *Ask the question.* It is important that you ask the question properly. To do this, it is best to write out the question before you begin your teaching. Do not say, "Give me some ideas about problems with medications"; rather, say, "What are some of the reasons that people do not take medications as prescribed by their doctors?" The first question is too vague and will result in all kinds of strange answers, whereas the second is geared specifically to finding out why people do not comply with medication regimes.

3. *Write down whatever the members of the group say.* Keep writing items until no more are generated. Do not stop to discuss items. Just clarify that you are writing down what the participants say. It is useful to have two people conducting a brainstorm: One monitors the group for responses while the other writes. If you are the only trainer, you might ask someone in the group to write for you. However, be sure that the person writes what is actually said, not his or her interpretation. The list of ideas will be easier to read if you use two different colors and alternate the colors of the responses.

4. *Ask if anyone needs clarification on what any of the items means.* Have the person originally offering the item give the clarification.

5. *Once all the items have been clarified, use the brainstorm material to summarize a point, begin a problem-solving session, or go on to further teaching or discussion.* For example, say you want to emphasize the advantages of exercise. Instead of giving a lecture, have the participants brainstorm all the advantages. Then you can correct any misconceptions or add the one or two things the group forgot. Another use of brainstorms is to solve problems. Let's say that someone in the group has a problem, such as not being able to avoid all the tempting food brought to work by coworkers. Instead of offering solutions yourself, ask the group for solutions. Then have the person with the problem indicate the one or two solutions he or she will try.

Role Playing

There are at least two reasons for using role playing in patient education. First, it allows participants to discuss issues that they might otherwise feel were too sensitive. Second, it allows participants to practice a new skill or rehearse for a future difficult situation. It should be noted that role playing is a difficult training skill and should be used only by a patient educator who is comfortable with the technique. Also, participants often feel threatened and therefore do not like to role-play. No one likes to be on display, especially if he or she might be made to look foolish. Several variations of role playing can help to control the situation and protect the participants.

Coaching. Give the participants a situation: For example, pretend that you are expressing dissatisfaction to your doctor. One person plays the doctor and one the patient. After the patient has expressed dissatisfaction, make some suggestion about how he or she might have done this differently, and then reenact the role play using your alternative. A variation on this is to ask members

of the group for suggestions on how they might change the interaction. Again, it is important that the person role-playing the patient practice whatever solution is chosen. A second variation is
to role-play in threes. The first person is the doctor, the second
the patient, and the third the coach. In this case, have three situations so that everyone has a chance to play each role.

In a third variation, the patient educator takes one of the
roles. For example, if a participant expresses difficulty in communicating with her child, the trainer takes the role of the child.
In this way, the trainer can be sure that the responses are not too
bizarre or threatening to the participant.

Group Role Plays. Here the trainer plays one role—for example, a
patient who is very concerned about surgery—and the whole
group plays the second role—for example, the nurse. First, one
person counsels the "patient," and if he or she gets stuck, someone else in the group takes over. This is a very nonthreatening
form of role playing and is easily controlled by the trainer.

Rehearsal. This is one of the most useful forms of role play. Give
the patient a situation that he or she might encounter: For example, a postcardiac patient on a low-calorie diet goes out to eat
with friends who urge her to have dessert. The patient can then
practice refusal skills. People who rehearse difficult situations
before actually encountering them do better when faced with
them in the real world. By the way, rehearsal can easily be combined with coaching or group role plays.

Questioning

Questioning is one of the most important of all patient education skills. Not only does it enable you to find out what the patient knows, it can also be a useful way of teaching new skills. A
basic rule for all questioning is that you should very seldom ask

questions that can be answered by a yes or a no. Open-ended questions are much better. Do not ask, "Are you feeling better today?" Ask, "How are you feeling today?"

The following are some ways that you might use questioning in your patient teaching:

- *The patient knows what he or she should do but is not doing it.* Ask, "Why do you smoke?" "What are you afraid might happen if you lost weight?" or "What problems do you think you might have in starting an exercise program?"
- *You are helping a patient solve a problem.* Ask, "What solutions do you see for this problem?" "Where might you go to get other ideas?" or "Which of these solutions would you like to try?" It is always better to teach problem-solving skills than to solve problems. Of course, in some situations, it is best to give an answer. If a patient asks which type of oil is low in cholesterol, there is no reason to cause frustration by telling him or her to go to the library.

One word of caution about questioning: Keep your voice tone neutral. Sometimes, when poorly asked, questions sound judgmental—for example, " *Why* do *you* smoke?" instead of " *Why* do you smoke?"

Appendix 4A at the end of this chapter contains a list of questions used as examples in this volume that you can ask patients to determine their needs, abilities, beliefs, and understanding.

Self-Monitoring

One of the best ways to get people to change behaviors is to let them monitor their own experience. People have a difficult time denying their own evidence. On the more positive side, self-monitoring helps a person see his or her problems or progress. Examples of self-monitoring include keeping a food diary or keeping track of when headaches occur. This information can then be used as the basis for behavior change. Self-monitoring can also be used as feedback, such as weekly weigh-ins and keeping track of exercise progress. This is like the feedback that is so important for obtaining skills mastery. For more on self-monitoring and skills mastery, see Chapter 2.

Creative patient educators can almost always build some self-monitoring techniques into their programs. The following are some concrete examples.

Diet

In many cases, patients are trying to change their diet—to lose weight, to lower cholesterol, to increase calcium, to decrease fats, or to conform to some regime such as a diabetic diet. In all these cases, a good place to start is to have patients keep a 4-day diet history in which they write down everything they eat as they eat it. The 4 days should probably be 2 weekend days and 2 weekdays. Fridays are more like weekend days than weekdays and thus should probably not be counted in the 4 days. This self-monitoring of food intake helps patients see where the problems lie and make plans to change. After being on a program for a while, they can again do a 4-day diary to see progress and check for any new problems. If 4 days seems too much, then 2 days will do, preferably a Sunday and Monday.

Exercise

There are several ways to monitor exercise. The time spent exercising, the distance covered, the weights lifted, and the number of repetitions all help people see how they are progressing. While exercising, patients can take their own pulse to be sure that they are in an aerobic zone. A quick self-monitoring test is that if they cannot talk while exercising (unless, of course, they are swimming), then they are exercising too hard. Such simple self-monitoring guidelines are helpful in getting people started and take some of the fear away about doing too much.

Diabetes

Blood glucose monitoring is a good way of helping a diabetic self-monitor. However, we must be cautious in always insisting on glucose monitoring. Many people may not be able to afford monitoring supplies. Although machines are low priced and readily available, the monthly purchase of supplies can be quite expensive. If a population does not have the means to afford glucose monitoring, it should be de-emphasized in diabetic teaching. Insisting that people do something they cannot afford to do only frustrates them and makes it more likely they will take no action to keep their blood glucose under control.

Hypertension

We know that many people have white-coat hypertension; that is, their blood pressure is much higher in the doctor's office than at any other time. Therefore, self-monitoring of blood pressure is very helpful. This can be done by getting patients to have their blood pressure taken regularly—perhaps at a supermarket that has a blood pressure machine, at a community health center, at the blood bank when giving blood, or at special events held during health awareness weeks such as National Health Week. You might even teach clients how to take their own blood pressure and have equipment available at a convenient location. It is not important that the readings be 100% accurate. Rather, patients can see how their blood pressure changes over time. Of course, they need a little instruction in the meaning of the numbers.

Weight Loss

Scales are wonderful self-monitoring devices.

Asthma

In the case of asthma, you are trying to teach symptom recognition as well as to get people to act on their symptoms before the symptoms become serious. Peak-flow meters are useful for this. Monitoring can include keeping track of the number of times one must call the doctor, go to the emergency room, or miss work because of asthma. Also, patients can keep track of when medication is taken and its relationship to the seriousness of the attack. Most important, you can teach patients the early warning signs of an asthma attack so that with watchful monitoring, attacks can be averted.

There are no doubt hundreds of other ways to help people self-monitor. The more of these that you can build into the program, the more chance you will have of seeing real behavior change.

Action Planning

Sometimes taking the first step is the most difficult part of behavior change. Action plans go a long way toward helping this situation and can also be used to establish and maintain new behaviors. The most important thing about an action plan is that it is something a patient chooses to do, not something that you, the health professional, insist that he or she does. An action plan not only gets the patient started with new behaviors, it helps to build the patient's confidence or self-efficacy. For more about action planning, see Appendix 4B as well as the section on self-efficacy in Chapter 2.

Problem Management

One of the most important skills for patients is problem management. Unfortunately, this is seldom formally taught in patient education programs. We teach problem management, rather than problem solving, because sometimes problems cannot be

solved. Life must be managed around them. It is okay to didacti-
cally introduce patients to the formal problem-solving steps:

1. Define the problem.
2. List possible solutions.
3. Pick a solution and try it.
4. Evaluate the results.
5. If necessary, try another solution.
6. If necessary, seek advice from others.
7. If necessary, accept that this may not be a problem that can be
   solved right now.

However, it is more important that patients be given an opportunity to practice problem management skills. When a problem arises, ask the patient what suggestions he or she has to solve
the problem. If there are other patients available, you can also
ask them for ideas. Finally, you can offer suggestions. Then ask
the patient to pick one of the suggestions to try.

This process not only teaches patients the problem management process, it teaches them that they can get ideas from other
patients, friends, and family members. They become active
problem managers rather than depending on health professionals to solve problems.

One note of caution: As health professionals, we have been
taught to solve problems. Helping patients to manage problems
is often, for us, a new skill. We need to be careful not to slip back
into our old, comfortable problem-solving behaviors.

¤ WHO WILL TEACH THE PROGRAM?

It is usually best to decide who is going to present your program before it is developed. In this way, you can include the presenters in program development. No one likes to be told to do

something when he or she has had no input. But sometimes, the program presenters are chosen only after the program is fully developed. This is especially true with very standardized programs.

We usually choose our teachers based on their expertise in subject matter, with little attention to their teaching skills or knowledge of patient education. Although it is important that the teacher have content knowledge, it is not necessary that he or she know everything about the subject. What is important is that he or she know the key messages and good patient education process. Often, laypersons with the disease can be excellent instructors, as can lay professional teams.

¤ KNOWING WHAT TO TEACH AND WHEN TO TEACH

Unfortunately, when working with patients one to one, very few health professionals give much thought as to what they should teach. There is just no time. Therefore, it is important that this decision process occur before the actual patient encounter. Thus, if a patient is in for bypass surgery, there should be a set protocol of things to teach. In fact, a checklist can be made up and then checked off as the patient education is delivered. The problem is not that professionals do not know the content. It is usually that they know too much and try to teach it all. To prove this yourself, try an experiment. Sit through any patient education program and count the number of things that patients are taught. I did this recently with a 5-week diabetes program and counted 127 messages, some of them unclear or contradictory. Is it a wonder our patients do not follow our instructions? (See Chapter 1 for information on how to select key messages.)

Another problem is that patient educators sometimes decide, wisely, that it is impossible to teach it all–and they therefore decide to teach nothing. In neither case are patient needs served. Again, what is needed is a priority-setting process that clarifies for all professionals what they should be teaching to any specific patient. Sometimes protocols or patient maps can be written that include what should be taught at each stage of the hospital stay: for example, preoperative, immediate postoperative, 2 or 3 days postoperative, and just before the patient leaves.

¤ KNOWING HOW TO TEACH

Most health professionals believe that they know how to teach. The reality is that most of us are only poor to fair patient educators. There are several reasons for this. First, few of us have had any formal training in patient education. Lacking this training, we try to emulate the teaching that we have received. The problem with this approach is that most school-type teaching is aimed at passing on knowledge. Patient education is aimed at changing behaviors or health status. Thus the teaching methods are different and must be learned and practiced.

In planning patient education programs, it is often necessary to teach patient education skills to the patient educators. These skills include the use of questioning, problem solving, goal setting, demonstration, and return demonstration. All of these are discussed earlier in this chapter. The important thing to note is that sometimes, preparing a program is not enough. Significant time and effort must be spent on preparing health professionals or laypersons to take on the role of successful patient educators.

Recently, we have seen a new type of physician-led group visits. These combine the medical encounter with patient education. Typically, a physician (sometimes helped by someone with group process skills) meets with his or her patients for approximately 2 hours. During this time, the doctor talks about a topic of interest to his patients, such as migraine headaches, or medical tests, answers questions, and talks with patients individually during break time to answer quick personal questions or write prescriptions. Finally, patients and the physician plan together for the next visit—usually in about a month. Group visits can have many forms, from drop-in visits to ongoing, diagnosis-specific visits to visits with patients who have mixed diagnoses. (For more about group visits, see Beck et al., 1997.)

¤ ONE-ON-ONE EDUCATION

One-on-one education is the most common type of patient education. It is what doctors, nurses, and other health professionals do at the bedside or in the clinic. In one-on-one education, there are four major considerations: time, knowing what to teach, knowing how to teach, and documenting what has been taught.

Time is an especially valuable commodity for doctors and, to a slightly lesser extent, for other health care professionals. Most doctors have only 10 to 20 minutes in which to interact with a patient. Therefore, any education must be very quick. Some have called these 30-second interventions. So what can you do in 30 seconds? A great deal. A doctor can tell a patient, "I want you to stop smoking." This is one of the most powerful things a doctor can do to get someone to stop smoking. When doing a breast examination, the doctor can ask the patient to demonstrate how she examines her breasts. It has been found that getting a woman to touch her own breast is one of the best ways of ensuring future breast self-examination. Patients receiving prescriptions should always be asked how they are going to take the medication. This simple question helps to reveal any problems or misunderstandings. For example, one patient I know, when given an antibiotic labeled "Avoid exposure to sunlight," was very careful to keep the pills in a dark place. She never considered that she should avoid exposure to sun herself. Finally, the doctor can make referrals: "I know that you want to lose weight; here is a list of resources in our community to help you with that effort." These are just a few of many possible 30-second interventions. In planning what you want doctors to do, it is important to be realistic.

Nurses, physiotherapists, occupational therapists, and other health professionals also have limited time. However, it may not be as limited as that of a doctor. Therefore, you might think of 3- to 5-minute interventions that can realistically take place in the context of normal practice. If you use some of the priority-setting techniques discussed earlier in this chapter, these few minutes can be well utilized. In all cases, it is important to separate out what a patient wants and needs to know from what the health professional wants to teach. The priority should always be on the former. Sometimes a compromise can be reached. If the patient is concerned about fatigue and you want to teach about diet, you can frame your teaching by explaining how fatigue is often due to poor diet and thus can be helped by your suggestions.

◘ GROUP EDUCATION

Everything that we have said about one-on-one education is also true for group education. The difference is that the patient educator must have a greater variety of skills. In addition to all the one-on-one skills mentioned above, the educator, if he or she is going to do more than just lecture, must have skills in group process. Again, you are not born with these skills but rather learn them from life experience or in a structured manner. A complete program for training patient educators is beyond the scope of this book. However, it is important to be aware of the possibility that you may need to train your patient educators or see that they receive training.

✪ SPECIAL PROBLEMS WITH GROUPS

When patients come to groups, they come for different reasons and have different knowledge and skill levels. This is true
no matter how specific you try to make your intake criteria.
Therefore, in any group setting, meeting the needs of the individual members is a problem. There are several ways of handling
this. First, make sure that all members know what to expect from
the course. You can do this by using a matrix needs assessment
(see Chapter 1). If you find that someone has needs that are very
different from those of the rest of the group, you can let him or
her know that this might not be the educational program for him
or her. The outliers then have the option of staying or not. If they
do stay, they will have no illusions about what the course will
cover.

Another way of dealing with differences is to have everyone
work on developing his or her own behavioral program. Thus, in
a class on lowering cholesterol, some people may choose to increase fiber, others to cut down on eggs and dairy products, and
still others to eat less red meat. When behaviors are flexible instead of prescriptive, they are much more likely to be meaningful (see the subsection above on determining which behaviors
are relatively easy to change).

Finally, people with more knowledge and skills can be utilized to help those with less background. They can help in problem solving and can sometimes also be used as successful coping
models (see Chapter 2 for a discussion of modeling). It is important that group education avoid being too rigid and prescriptive.
If it is flexible, the varied backgrounds of the participants become an advantage, not a problem.

A note of caution: The following often happens in groups
that I have observed. The instructor asks the group members
what questions or problems they have. If someone does not ask a
question in 5 seconds, the instructor assumes there are no ques-

tions and continues with a lecture. Sometimes, the instructor will wait a few more seconds, and someone will ask a question. The instructor then spends several minutes answering the question and goes on with the lecture without ever finding out if anyone else now has questions. After the class, the instructor says she has a very quiet group, never realizing that she does not give them a real chance to participate. In fact, if the group had been participating, she could not get in all of her lecture, visual aids, and demonstrations. Group participation does not just happen. Time must be planned for it, and it must be fostered.

✷ PUTTING IT ALL TOGETHER

So far, we have looked at many of the pieces that are necessary for putting together a patient education program. However, the real trick of patient education is putting the content and process together in a package that helps patients reach the outcome objectives. Such packaging usually takes the form of a protocol that outlines the general topics to be covered in the program. Good patient education protocols should also be so detailed that someone who is not familiar with the program can pick it up and replicate what you are doing. The reason that such detailed protocols are not usually done is that they require considerable thought and preparation.

In preparing a protocol, there are several things to keep in mind:

1. *Write your objectives and be sure that what you are teaching is designed to meet these objectives.* For example, if you want a cardiac patient to exercise, do not spend the majority of your time explaining disease process. If you want an intervention to be interactive, use as little lecture as possible and build in interactive activities. These do not just happen; they have to be planned.

2. *Look at your resources—time, personal, money, space.* What you find will help you choose, if you are planning a one-on-one intervention, a mediated intervention (one that uses audio, visual, or both types of materials), a one-time group meeting, a short course, or an ongoing support group. Do not assume that just because something has always been done one way, it cannot be done another way. For example, people with knee pain usually have one-on-one appointments with physical therapists. In one major health facility, knee classes for people with knee pain are held twice weekly. People can attend as often as they wish. There is no waiting for appointments or concern because of insurance limits. Experience has shown that after initial hesitation, both patients and physical therapists are happy with the new system.

3. *Make sure that you vary your activities.* Everyone gets tired of the same format. Thus you might include some lecture, brainstorming, a film, and general discussion all in one session. It is especially important to encourage active participation of group members after lunch or dinner because these are times that people sometimes get sluggish or are apt to fall asleep. A good time to introduce new activities is early in the day, when people are fresh. Another trick of the trade is to save some of your most interesting material until last. This encourages people to stay to the end instead of leaving early.

4. *No matter what intervention you choose, do not waste the first few minutes.* This is the most important part of the intervention and the place where you can least afford mistakes. In educational terms, this is called the *set.* It (a) lets participants meet each other, (b) tells them what to expect, and (c) lets them decide to participate. Note how Activity 1 in the chronic-disease workshop protocol given in Appendix 4B at the end of this chapter was designed to meet these objectives. First, participants name their disease and then tell about their major disease-related problems.

This lets everyone know a little about the others in the group. It also establishes the fact that there are common concerns. From a process point of view, it forces everyone to participate in a nonthreatening way. Because the workshop is very interactive, it is important to model expectations early. It is one thing to tell participants that a class is interactive and quite another to see that interaction really happens.

After everyone participates, there is a brief lecture about expectations, and then participants are given an overview of the course and shown how their concerns are specifically met by this course.

Please note that the original instructions, "Have all participants introduce themselves and share two or three of the biggest problems they have because of their chronic health problems," are very specific. We do not ask people to "tell a little about themselves" or to talk about their disease. If either of these was used as an opener, people would give long discourses that would take up much more than the allotted time.

The opening is also kept on track by having the leaders model the desired behavior. The group will almost always follow the example of the first person. Therefore, it is important to set a good example.

5. *If at all possible, build on activities over several weeks.* Thus, rather than having one session on diet and another on exercise, have two or more sessions that include or add to both of these subjects. In this way, participants will have a chance to go home, decide what they want to do, try things out, and report back with problems. Then there is still time to make changes.

6. *Try to use the same instructor or facilitator for every session.* This builds in continuity and helps to create rapport between the instructor and the participants, which is especially important for group education. If you use a different expert every session, this is not patient education but a lecture series; it is important to

understand that it is very unlikely that such a series will result in behavior change. However, lecture series are usually very good for increasing knowledge.

7. *Consider using a* Sesame Street *approach.* Much of traditional patient education is taught by topic. In the first week, we discuss exercise; in the next week, nutrition; in the third week, medications; and so on. No other education is carried out in this way. We usually have small doses of several topics, all of which are built on over time. This is what *Sesame Street* does. On each show, there are several segments. Each segment is then built upon each day. If you look at the topics discussed in the Chronic Disease Self-Management Program protocol in Appendix 4B, you will see that exercise is discussed in two out of six sessions and that feedback and action planning are part of every session. All sessions discuss four or five topics. The advantage of this approach is that people are not overwhelmed with new material. They have a chance to try new activities, to come back and make corrections, and then to add to their program. The disadvantage is that you cannot have a different expert talk at each session.

8. *Use ritual.* There is security for both instructors and students in a known structure. This is one of the reasons Alcoholics Anonymous and other 12-step programs are so successful. By ritual, we mean structure: Each class has a defined beginning, middle, and end that look much the same, session after session. In our Chronic Disease Self-Management Program protocol example (Appendix 4B), each class starts with feedback and ends with action planning. Structure helps to set group norms and expectations. It is one of the things that can be used to strengthen an intervention at no extra cost in time, money, or materials.

9. *Frame your teaching around patient needs and beliefs.* For example, topics could include pain management, dealing with anger, and beating fatigue rather than the use of medication, coping, and exercise. Note that the same material is taught, but in different ways. (For more about framing, see Chapter 7.)

10. *Do not try to change patient beliefs or practices unless they are causing harm.* If patients want to drink vinegar and honey, it probably will not hurt them. It is easier to add to beliefs than to change or destroy them.

11. *Be consistent with your messages.* If you are teaching self-management, then make patients responsible for finding information or making copies of materials. You cannot teach self-management and then manage for the patient.

12. *Remember that patients always have choices.* Often, many activities will accomplish the same end. Patients always have the option of not doing what you suggest. There are two lessons here. First, do not be dogmatic. Second, remind patients that the decisions and choices are theirs.

13. *Do not try to crowd everything into whatever time you have.* The most common mistake in patient education is trying to include too much. In our need to give information, we often give up using the processes that make the information useful. Be very selective about what you teach. Everything that happens should be directly related to the objectives. You can always give your clients written material if they want more information.

(One important note: Patients will often ask many questions or become argumentative to avoid taking action. This is especially true in a class situation. To avoid this, tell any person who becomes argumentative that you will talk with him or her during break or after class.)

14. *Do not spend a lot of time with one person.* If you do, you probably will not help that person and will definitely ensure that the others in your group who may be more ready to make changes will not be helped.

15. *Give attention for taking positive action.* All too often, we spend our time trying to convince people to do something they have no intention of doing. They like the attention they get for not doing things. It is hard, but the best strategy is to help those who want help. For those who do not want to get down to

business, remind them that it is their choice (see point 9, above). When those who are hesitant to act see others who are successful and when they do not get rewarded for inaction, there is a good chance that they will begin to manage their condition.

Appendix 4B at the end of this chapter is the protocol for the first session of the Chronic Disease Self-Management Program. For more information on this program, see the Stanford Patient Education Research Center Web site at http://www.stanford. edu/group/perc/perchome.html.

¤ DISSEMINATION

In the past, patient educators were responsible for developing programs that were carried out by only a few people in one institution. Even programs that had been demonstrated to be efficacious were often not disseminated beyond the developers' home institution. This is no longer the case. As our health systems increase in size and complexity, it is important that we design programs that can be easily replicated throughout a health care system. In addition, for programs to be sustainable, they must be shown to improve health status and, if possible, to lower health care costs. Unfortunately, we do not know a great deal about how to ensure that a program will be disseminated. The following, however, are some suggestions based on our own experience and that of others.

Protocol

If you want a program to be used by others, its protocol must be written in such a way that others can read the directions and follow them. For example, in a cardiac program, it is not enough to write, "Lecture about aerobic exercise" or even to give an outline of the lecture. Rather, every detail of both content and process must be written. Writing a good protocol is like writing a good recipe. If the details are lacking, then the quality of the product is not assured. For an example of a protocol, see Appendix 4B.

Evaluation

More and more health care systems are looking for patient education programs that have been proven to be efficacious. This means that you should evaluate your program and be prepared to share the results. Some suggestions on evaluation are found in Chapter 3. Unfortunately, some patient educators conduct evaluations and then do not use the results. In some cases, they find that their programs are not doing much to assist their patients. This is a good reason to look at your program and change it to be more effective. Sometimes, however, educators do not want to believe the results of their own evaluations and just ignore the results. In medicine, new drugs must first be shown to do no harm and then must demonstrate that they are at least as effective as similar existing treatments. Although patient education does not yet have to meet these standards, it may be well for us to consider them when deciding how to use the results of our evaluations.

In some cases, evaluation shows that a program is efficacious, but this is as far as it goes. The results are never published or shared. The reasons for this are many. Maybe the patient educators are unsure about how to write up a study, or maybe other health professionals have been discouraging because the study design is not "clean" enough. More often, there is not enough time, and other things take priority. Unfortunately, these are the reasons that some of our most important knowledge is lost.

Publishing

Many practitioners feel that only academics publish. This is not true. If you have a good program and want others to share it, you must publish. Somehow, in the health care world of today, the results of an evaluation are not considered real until they are published. This is sometimes a slow and tedious process, but is well worth the effort. You do not have to publish in a major medical journal, although that would be nice. Rather, look at clinical practice journals within your field, such as *Diabetes Educator* and *Arthritis Care and Research*. You can also look toward professional journals such as *Health Education Behavior* and *Patient Education and Counseling*. Both of these journals accept practice articles that do not have to adhere to the more rigorous standards of research articles.

Submitting an article need not be a mysterious process. First, find the journal to which you want to submit. In every issue, there is usually a page that gives instructions to authors. Follow those instructions exactly. After you submit your article, the journal's editor will usually send it to two or three reviewers. These are usually people who have published in the journal and are familiar with the topic. Sometimes these reviews are blind—that is, they do not know who wrote the article. Other journals do not blind their reviewers. In no case will you know who reviewed your article.

The reviewers then send their comments back to the editor, who makes a decision to publish the article, reject the article, or ask you to rewrite the article. The decision, along with the reviews, is sent to you. Reviewing the reviews is almost always a traumatic time. It is very rare for an article to get accepted the first time it is submitted. If the editor asks for a rewrite, do it; just be sure to include all of the suggestions made by the reviewers in that rewrite. If this is not possible, explain why. When an editor asks for a rewrite, it usually means that your article will be accepted if you do what he or she wants. Be warned, however, that your article can be rejected even after a rewrite.

If the article is rejected, read the comments of the reviewers and do whatever you do when you are angry. Put the comments away for a week or two and then read them again. Use the comments when you rewrite the article to submit it to another journal. Unfortunately, many good patient education studies are lost because the authors are not persistent. It is my experience that it usually takes one rejection and one or two rewrites before an article is published. This process often takes 2 or more years. Before deciding that publishing is too much trouble, consider that this is one of the best ways to assure acceptance and dissemination of your program.

Professional Meetings

Take every opportunity you can to talk about your program at professional meetings. If you are invited to speak, say yes. When it is appropriate, submit abstracts. These meetings do not have to be large national affairs. Rather, you might talk to the monthly PT staff meeting or the weekly meeting of the medical staff. The more people who know about your program and support it, the more likely it is to be disseminated.

Cultivate a Champion

A champion is someone in your organization who both supports your program and is an opinion leader—a person who is respected and listened to by others. Champions for patient education programs are often, but not always, physicians. If at all possible, the time to find a champion is not when your program is complete but when you start working on it. The champion should have an integral part in planning and conducting your program. In this way, the program becomes your champion's program, and he or she is more apt to support it. For example, when we were first developing the Chronic Disease Self-Management Program, we involved the physician who is the director of health education for a major health maintenance organization. He was involved in every phase of the program, from writing some of the patient materials to developing the evaluation scheme. He was also helpful in recruiting patients. Because of this early involvement, it was an easy step for him to become a champion for the program within his own organization and also a representative of the program at national meetings. Champions do not just appear; you must create and nurture them.

One caution about cultivating a champion: Often, you may find a physician or other health professional who is very enthusiastic about your program but is not well established with his or her peers. This may be a young professional or someone who is very interested in alternative medicine. Such an individual can be very helpful in the development of your program and program materials, but he or she may be counterproductive in the role of champion. A champion must be someone who is already well established and respected within his or her own profession.

✪ APPENDIX 4A: QUESTIONS IN PATIENT EDUCATION
(with thanks to Mary Hobb, MPH)

Asking good questions is your best means of determining a patient's needs, abilities, beliefs, and understanding. It is a key to excellence in patient education.

In general, use open-ended questions to elicit a meaningful response; avoid questions that can be answered with yes or no. Use a neutral, not judgmental, voice. For example:

Yes-No Question	*Open-Ended Question*
Are you feeling better today?	How are you feeling today?
Do you know why you should quit smoking?	Why do you smoke?
Are you going to start exercising?	What problems do you think you might have in starting an exercise program?
Can you cut back on meat?	What will be your biggest problem with cutting down on the amount of meat you are eating?
Do you have any questions?	What questions do you have?

The following is a list of additional questions from this book for your easy reference:

1. Questions on salient beliefs to give you insight into the patient's beliefs and concerns about a particular condition or behavior:
   - When you think of _____ (e.g., diabetes, exercise), what do you think of?
   - What would you do if _____?

2. Needs assessment questions to determine priorities for teaching:
   - What are your greatest problems in living with _____ (heart disease, a low-fat diet)?
   - Which changes would you like to start on? (give the patient a list of changes you are recommending, e.g., exercise, low-fat diet, quitting smoking, controlling stress, losing weight)
   - If you _____ (stop smoking, start exercising, etc.), what are you afraid might happen?
   - What do you think causes _____ (pain, diabetes, etc.)?
   - Why is exercise important to you?
   - Why don't you _____?

3. Questions to determine cultural issues that could affect health behavior:
   - When you hear the word _____ (diabetes, stomach problem, etc.) what do you think about?
   - What will make it better?
   - What do you expect me to do for you?
4. Questions to check for understanding (ask patients to repeat back what they understand):
   - So how much are you going to walk tomorrow after you are home?
5. Self-efficacy questions to determine likelihood of success:
   - On a scale of 1 to 10, how sure are you that you can do _____ (a very specific behavior, such as walking for 15 minutes, 3 times a week)? (If the patient's answer is 7 or less, ask him or her to revise the goal to ensure success.)
6. Questions to test the likelihood of compliance:
   - What problems do you expect in _____ (exercising, taking medications)?
7. Questions to reinforce a new behavior:
   - Role play: "Okay, say I'm your friend and you are you, and we are at a party and I am encouraging you to eat a piece of fried chicken. How would you say 'no thanks' to me?"

◻ APPENDIX 4B: PROTOCOL FOR THE FIRST SESSION OF THE CHRONIC DISEASE SELF-MANAGEMENT WORKSHOP

The following is the protocol from the first 2.5-hour session of the Chronic Disease Self-Management Workshop (Lorig et al., 1999). This patient education program is offered in many parts of the United States, Australia, New Zealand, Canada, Norway, Holland, and Hong Kong. The course is designed to be taught by a pair of leaders, at least one of whom is a layperson with a chronic illness. Self-efficacy theory serves as the theoretical framework for the course. As you read over this protocol, note that the session has specific objectives and that the activities are varied, starting with an interactive exercise. Activity 1 sets the tone for the following 13.5 hours. It clearly sets forth the expectations for the group's participation by reviewing the class guidelines (Chart 2). Also, within the first few minutes, there is a course overview (Chart 1) that helps participants decide if they have come to the right course.

Activity 2 reinforces this tone with a brief lecture on self-help principles in the context of chronic disease.

Activity 3 is an example of helping participants to reinterpret physiological signs and symptoms. This is one of the ways to enhance self-efficacy (see Chapter 2).

Activity 4 is an introduction to how symptoms interrelate and then focuses on an introduction to cognitive techniques that can be used to break the symptom cycle.

Activity 5 is an introduction to action plans. Note that this activity uses both lecture and participation.

Activity 6 is the ending for every class. Action planning is used to assist participants in gaining skills mastery. This is another important component for building self-efficacy.

In summary, this 2.5-hour session uses several educational processes, including the group's sharing of experience, lecture, visual charts, brainstorming, an experiential exercise, and action planning. In addition, it covers several content areas, including a needs assessment, discussion of disease process, and introduction to cognitive symptom management. In short, this first session sets the stage for the use of content and process for the entire 13.5 hours.

Chronic Disease Self-Management Workshop: Session 1 (© 1999 Stanford University; reprinted by permission)

Purpose

- To introduce the group members to each other
- To inform the group about the general principles of self-management
- To identify the group members' problems caused by chronic illness
- To differentiate chronic illness from acute disease
- To identify and emphasize the common elements of various chronic health problems
- To introduce the cause of discomfort
- To introduce cognitive symptom management techniques
- To introduce action plans as a key self-management tool

Objectives

By the end of this session, the group members will be able to

1. Define at least three differences between acute and chronic disease
2. Identify a set of problems that are common among various chronic illnesses
3. Identify the components of the symptom cycle
4. Name at least two cognitive symptom management techniques
5. Make a self-management behavior action plan for the coming week

Materials

- **Charts 1-6**
- Blank name tags for everyone (these should be reusable, as you will need them every week)

- Easel
- Blank flip charts/felt pens or blackboard chalk
- *Living a Healthy Life With Chronic Conditions* for each household
- Pad of paper, extra pencils
- Kleenex

Agenda (Post this agenda)

- Activity 1: Introduction–Identifying Common Problems (*30 minutes*)
- Activity 2: Workshop Overview and Responsibilities (*10 minutes*)
- Activity 3: Differences Between Acute and Chronic Conditions (*15 minutes*)
- **Break** (*20 minutes*)
- Activity 4: Introduction to Cognitive Symptom Management (*15 minutes*)
- Activity 5: Introduction to Action Plans (*40 minutes*)
- Activity 6: Closing (*10 minutes*)

Activity 1: Introduction (30 minutes)

Methods

- Lecturette
- Group introductions

Note: Charts for this workshop are shown in boxes throughout this manual. The material printed in the boxes *in italics* may be added verbally and need not be printed on the charts. Only the material printed **in bold** needs to be printed on the charts.

1. As participants arrive, *distribute name tags*. Have them write the names they like to be called (first name or nickname, not last name). These should be large enough so that they can be read from across the room. Felt pens are good for this.

2. **Welcome** the group and explain that you will all be introducing yourselves and stating your chronic health condition(s) and what problems the chronic health problem has caused you.

   Introduce yourself. In your introduction, name any chronic illness you have and name two or three problems you have because of your health condition. Be careful with your introduction as **you will be modeling** how the participants will introduce themselves. (Modeling will be important for every activity you do. Leaders should *always model* the activity *before* asking the participant to do so.) Do not dwell on your specific problem(s). The introduction might be something like this: "I'm John Doe and I have emphysema. This has meant slowing down and never being sure how I will feel day to day."

   > IMPORTANT MODELING MOMENT

3. **Group introductions.** Have all participants introduce themselves and share **two or three of the biggest problems** they have because of their chronic health problems. Do not let participants dwell on their specific condition or symptoms. If this happens, remind them that what you want them to share are a couple of *problems* they have *because* of their illness, and that they do not need to go into a lot of detail.

   People **without** chronic conditions should share problems **they** have that are caused by living with someone with chronic health problems.

   One leader should be leading the activity while the other is listing the problems on the board or chartpad. Put a check mark next to each problem as it is mentioned after the first time.

4. Point out that even though they have different chronic health conditions, many of their concerns are the same.

Activity 2: Workshop Overview and Responsibilities (10 minutes)

Methods

- Lecturette

1. Using **Chart 1,** give an overview of the workshop. Emphasize how the content relates to the problems that the group just identified. Refer back to their list of problems on the board or chartpad.

If participants indicate interest in topics that will not be addressed (such as surgery or research), state that they can proba-

Chart 1 Workshop Overview

	Week 1	Week 2	Week 3	Week 4	Week 5	Week 6
Overview of self-management and chronic conditions	✔					
Making an action plan	✔	✔	✔	✔	✔	✔
Relaxation/cognitive symptom management	✔		✔	✔	✔	✔
Feedback/problem-solving		✔	✔	✔	✔	✔
Anger/fear/frustration		✔				
Fitness/exercise		✔	✔			
Better breathing			✔			
Fatigue			✔			
Nutrition				✔		
Advance directives				✔		
Communication				✔		
Medications					✔	
Making treatment decisions					✔	
Depression					✔	
Informing the health care team						✔
Working with your health care professional						✔
Future plans						✔

bly find this information by calling the different disease-specific voluntary organizations, such as the American Heart Association, the American Lung Association, or the Arthritis Foundation. There may also be information in *Living a Healthy Life*.

2. Describe the responsibilities of the group (refer to **Chart 2**).

Chart 2 Responsibilities

---

1. **Come every session.**
2. **Ask anything you want.** *(If we don't know the answer, we will get it. Also, if time is short, we may ask you to hold your questions for later.)*
3. **Maintain confidentiality.** *(What is said in the group stays in the group.)*
4. **Do your homework.** *(It won't be graded, but it will make the workshop more valuable to you.)*
5. **Give new activities at least a 2-week trial** *(before deciding what will work best for you).*
6. **Make and complete a weekly action plan.** *(We will be talking more about this at the end of this session.)*
7. **Call your buddy weekly.** *(The leaders will call the first week. After that, you will need to find a buddy and call each other.)*

Activity 3: Differences Between Acute and Chronic Conditions (15 Minutes)

Methods

• Lecturette

Preparatory Reading

• *Living a Healthy Life,* Chapter 1

1. Refer to chart on page 3 of *Living a Healthy Life* to discuss the differences between acute and chronic illness.

2. **Lecturette** (paraphrase the following): Most of us think of our lives as a path. This path may have twists, turns, obstacles, and surprises. Having a chronic health problem changes the nature

of this path. As we indicated in our introduction, it brings about limitations, frustrations, and uncertainty about the future.

We can respond to these changes in many ways. For example, we can choose to do nothing and gradually lose the ability to do the things we wish, or we can work on improving or maintaining our overall fitness in order to maintain or regain some of our former pleasures. No matter what we do, we are managing our chronic health problem. Our choice is to be a passive manager of an active manager. If the choice is to actively manage, then we must be willing to take on three sets of self-management tasks (**Chart 3**).

Chart 3 Self-Management Tasks

---

1. **Take care of your health problem** *(such as taking medicine, exercising, going to the doctor, or changing diet).*
2. **Carry out your normal activities** (chores, employment, social life, etc.).
3. **Manage your emotional changes** *(changes brought about by your illness, such as anger, uncertainty about the future, changed expectations and goals, and sometimes depression. Changes can also happen in your relationships with family and friends).*

---

3. **Lecturette** (paraphrase the following): This workshop is aimed at teaching the self-management skills that will help us take on these tasks and enable us to shape our life path.

4. **Lecturette** (paraphrase the following): Being responsible for our condition includes the following:

   a. Keeping informed about our status—asking questions, reading, and so on.

   b. Taking part in planning out our treatment program by monitoring and reporting on our condition and sharing our preferences and goals with the physician and other members of the health care team.

   c. Maintaining the things in life that are meaningful to us. This may mean adapting the way we do things. For example, using a garden stool on wheels or having prepared dinners in the freezer for times that we are not feeling up to cooking.

d. Realizing that there will be emotional ups and downs and that the down parts are not pits to crawl out of but natural ups and downs that all paths have.

e. Seeking help and informing others about problems and changes we make in our daily program.

f. Setting goals and working toward them.

BREAK (20 minutes)

Activity 4: Introduction to Cognitive System Management (15 Minutes)

Methods

• Lecturette

• Demonstration

Preparatory Reading

• *Living a Healthy Life,* Chapter 6

1. **Using Chart 4, paraphrase the following lecturette:**

   Lecturette: We've all heard about the mind-body connection. We know that it has a significant impact on our body.

   Many people assume that the symptoms they are experiencing are due to only one cause: the disease. Although the disease can certainly cause pain, shortness of breath, fatigue, and so on, it is not the only cause. All these things in the cycle contribute to symptoms, and all can make them worse. Worse yet, they can feed on each other. Depression causes fatigue, stress causes tense muscles, and so on. This becomes a vicious cycle that gets worse and worse unless we find a way to break the cycle. By understanding how these things contribute to increased symptoms, we can learn techniques that help break the cycle at these various points. By using our minds to manage our stress, depression, and negative emotions, we have the first tool to help us feel better.

Chart 4

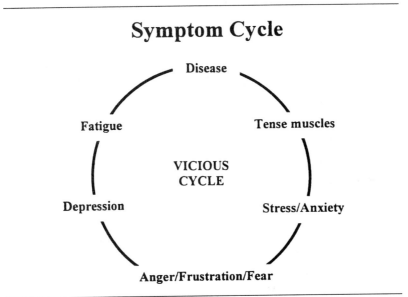

Symptom Cycle

Disease

Fatigue

Tense muscles

VICIOUS CYCLE

Depression

Stress/Anxiety

Anger/Frustration/Fear

2. To demonstrate the power of the mind, *ask the participants to do the following:*

Close your eyes and think about a bright yellow, juicy, ripe, lemon. You can smell its citrus aroma. Then imagine biting into the lemon, with the sour juice squirting into your mouth and dribbling down your chin. Suck the juice!

Give them a few seconds to imagine it, then ask them what happened. Point out that the salivation and puckering they experienced was solely due to their mind. There was no lemon present! This is a simple example of how the mind can affect the body. If we can affect the body so easily without trying very hard, imagine what we could accomplish if we worked at it!

3. **Lecturette** (paraphrase the following): There are many ways of using our minds to help manage such things as pain, discomfort

and fatigue. These techniques are generally called **cognitive techniques,** because they involve using the brain and cognitive or thinking type activities. In this workshop, we will learn several of these techniques. Our job is to try the various cognitive methods and find the ones that work best for us. Most people find that they like some techniques better than others.

4. **Lecturette** (paraphrase the following): Caution: *None of these techniques should be used to overcome chest pain.* This is a warning sign and should be managed in the way suggested by a physician.

5. **Chart 5** lists the various types of techniques:

Chart 5 Cognitive Symptom Management Methods

1. **Muscle relaxation** *(we will be doing this later in the workshop—it is a combination physical and cognitive technique)*

2. **Self-talk** *(looking at the ways we talk to ourselves and then changing the conversation—we will practice this later in the workshop, also)*

3. **Distraction** *(using our minds to think of something else—we will be trying this, too)*

4. **Guided Imagery** *(imagining ourselves in a story told by someone else—another technique we will learn)*

5. **Visualization** *(we tell ourselves a story or picture of ourselves achieving a goal—we will not do this, but there is a sample script in the book)*

6. **Lecturette** (paraphrase the following): Diaphragmatic breathing is another technique that we will be practicing. It can be used by itself to help relax and is often an important part of some of these cognitive techniques.

Activity 5: Introduction to Action Plans (40 minutes)

Methods

- Lecturette
- Participation

Preparatory Reading

- *Living a Healthy Life,* Chapter 2

1. **Lecturette** (paraphrase the following): One of the most important self-management skills is **goal setting.** It is an intermediate destination on your path. If we don't know where we are going, there is little chance that we will get there. For this workshop, we think of a goal as something we would like to accomplish in the next 3 to 6 months, such as being able to walk a half mile, visit the grandchildren, or socialize with friends. Take a moment now and **think of one or two goals.**

2. **Lecturette** (paraphrase the following): Goals are generally too big to work on all at once. Therefore, to achieve a goal, it needs to be broken down into smaller, more doable steps or tasks. For example, a person whose goal is to improve fitness might break into some of these steps at first: deciding what type of exercise to do, researching warm-water swimming pools or adaptive physical education classes at the community college, determining at what level he or she can exercise comfortably, reading about exercise in the *Living a Healthy Life* book, or finding a friend to exercise with.

3. **Lecturette** (paraphrase the following): Next, we need to get started by deciding which step we are going to work on **this week** and exactly how we are going to do it. This is done by making a **weekly action plan.** Review **Chart 6:**

Chart 6 Parts of an Action Plan

---

1. **Something YOU want to do** *(not what someone else thinks you should do or what you think you should do)*

2. **Reasonable** *(something you can expect to be able to accomplish this week)*

3. **Behavior-specific** *(for example, losing weight is not a behavior, but avoiding snacks between meals is a behavior)*

4. **Answer the questions:**

   What? *(for example, walking or avoiding snacks)*
   How much? *(for example, walking four blocks)*
   When? *(for example, after dinner or on Monday, Wednesday, Friday)*
   How often? *(for example, four times)*

5. **Confidence level of 7 or more** *(that you will complete the ENTIRE action plan)*

4. **PREPARE BEFORE SESSION:** Leaders should prepare action plans in advance with each other, remembering that the leaders' action plans will be **MODELS** for the rest of the participants. Leaders' action plans should be around behaviors taught in the workshop (e.g., exercise or relaxation techniques) and be realistic to the participants. Leaders should make action plans that are different; for example, one might be about exercise, and one might be about relaxation. Be careful that you make the action plan for 3-4 times a week, for example, rather than 5-7. **Practice** making your action plans with each other in the same way participants are asked to do:

5. Leader "A" asks Leader "B" what his or her action plan will be for this week. Leader "B" states his or her action plan, and Leader "A" asks Leader "B" what confidence level he or she has about completing the entire action plan (following the action plan script provided). Leaders then switch roles, with the Leader "A" giving his or her action plan. Then point out that the behavior, amount to be done, and when it will happen are all *very specific*.

> IMPORTANT
> MODELING
> MOMENT

6. Emphasize that action plans must be

   • something the person **wants to do**

   • **reasonable,** that is the person can expect to achieve it in the next week

7. Have participants break into pairs. **People with chronic health problems should pair up with people with chronic health problems, and significant others should pair up with significant others. Family members should *not* pair with each other.** Each pair helps each other make action plans just as the leaders did. *Each participant will report the action plan back to the entire group* after 10 minutes. Announce to the group after 4 minutes that they will switch with each other in one minute; announce that they should switch at 5 minutes; announce that they have one more minute at 9 minutes.

8. Reconvene the group. Ask participants to write their action plans down. An example of an action plan form can be found on pp. 20-21 of *Living a Healthy Life*. Participants may wish to

photocopy the form for use in the workshop, but *leaders are NOT to offer to photocopy the form for them!* (This is a self-management workshop.)

9. Ask for a volunteer to start reporting action plans and then go around the room from that person (do not ask for a second volunteer). Have participants report their action plans and *tell how confident* they are that they can accomplish it (10 is *very confident*, 0 is *not at all confident*). Emphasize that this number is *not* the percentage of the action plan they believe they can complete but how confident they are that they can complete the *whole* action plan. **If 7 or less,** problem-solve around the barriers causing the low confidence level and suggest that the participant adjust the action plan. (To help people make an action plan, refer to the action plan script below.)

   If someone is having trouble writing a clear action plan (i.e., specific activity, times per day, days per week), ask other group members for suggestions *before* you help. Do not spend more than 3 minutes with any one person. If someone is having problems, work with him or her individually *afterwards.*

10. Inform the participants that the *leaders will be calling them* once during the coming week to support them in their action plans.

Action Plan Script

I. Deciding what one wants to accomplish

Ask the person, "What will you do this week?" It is important that the activity come from the participant and not you. This activity does not have to be something covered in the workshop—just something that the participant wants to do to change behavior. Do not let anyone say, "I will try . . ." Each person should say, "I will . . ."

II. Making a plan

This is the difficult and most important part of making an action plan. Part I is worthless without Part II.

This plan should contain the following elements:

1. Exactly what is the participant going to do (i.e., how far will you walk, how will you eat less, what relaxation techniques will you practice)?

2. How much (i.e., walk around the block, 15 minutes, etc.)?

3. When will the participant do this? Again, this must be specific (i.e., before lunch, in the shower, when I come home from work).

4. How often will the activity be done? This is a bit tricky. Most participants tend to say every day. In making an action plan, the most important thing is to succeed. Therefore, it is better to commit to do something 4 times a week and exceed the commitment by actually doing it 5 times than to commit to do something every day and fail by only doing it 6 days. To ensure success, we usually encourage people to commit to do something 3 to 5 days a week. Remember that success and self-efficacy are as important, or maybe even more important, than actually doing the behavior.

III. Checking the action plan

Once the action plan is complete, ask the participant, "Given a scale of 0 to 10, with 0 being not at all confident and 10 being totally confident, how confident are you that you will (repeat the participant's action plan verbatim)?"

If the answer is 7 or above, this is probably a realistic action plan, and the participant would write it on his or her action plan/contract sheet.

If the answer is below 7, then the action plan should be reassessed. Ask the participant: "What makes you uncertain? What problems do you foresee?" Then discuss the problems. Ask other participants to offer solutions. YOU should offer solutions LAST. Once the problem-solving is completed, have the participant restate the action plan and return to repeat Part III, checking the action plan.

NOTE: This planning process may seem cumbersome and time-consuming. However, it does work and is well worth the effort. The first time you make action plans with a group, plan 2-3 minutes per person. Making an action plan is a learned skill. Your participant will soon be saying, "I will _____ four times this week before lunch and have a confidence level of 8 that I can do this." Thus, after two or three planning sessions, making an action should take less than a minute per participant.

Activity 6: Closing (6 minutes)

1. Invite participants to review what was covered today in **Chapters 1, 2, and 6** of *Living a Healthy Life*. Explain that this book is a reference book, not a syllabus. The workshop does not follow the book in order.

2. Remind participants to **keep track of their action plans** daily and bring them next week.

3. Remind participants that the **leaders will be calling them** during the week.

4. **Role play** a phone call, with one leader being the participant, according to the note to leaders below.

Note to Leaders

When making phone calls to participants, **BE BRIEF.** Split up the attendance list, each leader calling half of the participants.

"Hi, this is Jane from the Chronic Disease Self-Management Workshop. How are you doing with your action plan for walking this week?"

"My action plan is to swim three times a week. I have done it twice so far, so things are going well."

"I'm looking forward to hearing about your success."

5. Inform participants that we will begin to discuss exercise next week, as well as problem-solving and ways to deal with frustration, anger and fear.

6. Ask participants to bring their books each week.

7. Thank everyone for coming and collect the name tags.

8. Stay around for 15 minutes or so to answer questions and straighten up the room.

✿ BIBLIOGRAPHY

Beck, A., Scott, J., Williams, P., Robertson, B., Jackson, D., Gade, G., & Cowan, P. (1997). A randomized trial of group outpatient visits for chronically ill older HMO members: The Cooperative Health Care Clinic [see comments]. *Journal of the American Geriatrics Society, 45,* 543-549.

Ferguson, T., & Madara, E. J. (1996). *Health online: How to find health information, support groups, and self-help communities in cyberspace.* New York: Perseus.

Lorig, K., Holman, H., Sobel, D., Laurent, D., González, V., & Minor, M. (2000). *Living a healthy life with chronic conditions.* Palo Alto, CA: Bull Publishing.

Lorig, K., Sobel, D. S., Stewart, A. L., Brown, B. W., Jr., Bandura, A., Ritter, P., González, V. M., Laurent, D. D., & Homan, H. R. (1999). Evidence suggesting that a chronic disease self-management program can improve health status while reducing hospitalization: A randomized trial. *Medical Care, 37,* 5-14.

Mager, R. F. (1970). *Preparing instructional objectives.* Belmont, CA: Fearon.

Maxwell, B. (1998). *How to find health information on the Internet.* Washington, DC: Congressional Quarterly Books.

5

How Do I Get People to Come?

Virginia M. González
Kate Lorig

The best patient education program in the world does no one any good if no one comes. Low attendance can occur for many reasons. You may have created a product no one wants, people may not know about your program, your product may not be attractive, there may be factors that inhibit people from coming, or people may be actively discouraged from attending. In this chapter, we examine ways of marketing your program to health professionals, patients, and special populations who are hard to reach. Finally, we discuss some ways to use community resources to enhance your programs.

143

◘ MARKETING TO HEALTH PROFESSIONALS

Probably the strongest potential allies in marketing your program are other health professionals. At best, they can be very helpful. To be successful, you want to be sure that they are at least neutral. At worst, other professionals can completely destroy the program. With this in mind, let us start by examining how to get support from doctors and other health professionals. The time to start your marketing is when you plan your program. In Chapter 1, we talked about interested-parties analysis; this is a good technique to involve health professionals.

With health professionals, it is important not only to get their input but to let them be partners in the creation of your program. This does not mean endless group meetings. Rather, when you write content that would be of interest to a doctor, a physical therapist, or a nurse, have two or three key health professionals review it. Have a physician, a nurse, and a physical therapist review the whole program, offer comments, and suggest changes. In choosing your reviewers, do not just choose your friends. Rather, look for opinion leaders, health professionals who are highly respected by their peers. These might be instructors in health professional programs, officers in professional organizations, or senior, well-liked doctors. If your community has factions—for example, two hospitals—then choose reviewers from each faction.

Not only do you want health professionals as reviewers, you want to give these people ownership of the program. Ask if you can use their names on handouts or in publicity. When you write to other health professionals about the program, see if your reviewers will cosign your letter. A program invented by Howard Doe, R.N.; Helen Doe, M.D., Chief of Medicine; and Robin Doe, R.P.T, Director of Rehabilitation, may be easily introduced because it comes from credible sources.

Anyone who has ever invented anything has come across the dreaded NIH (not invented here) syndrome. You will recognize the symptoms when you hear "That may be the way they do it in New Zealand but not here in Australia"; "Those people in California just do not understand our health system"; or "People here are different." The quickest way to defuse this situation is to ask the "locals" to review the program and work with them to make any specific local adaptations. This forces the locals to look carefully at the program, rather than disliking it from afar. The revisions they make are usually very minor and may even help market the program locally. Most important of all, the local professionals now have ownership of the course, so NIH becomes IH—that is, "invented here."

A second problem we often hear is, "We cannot get doctors and other health professionals to refer people to our programs." If you survive the NIH syndrome, then the problem is probably that your professionals forget, find making a referral too complicated, or just do not have the time. As one physician told me, "It is not part of my dance." Today, most health professionals are very busy. They have very little time and must prioritize what they tell patients. Most do not have adequate time to provide a diagnosis and treatment. Therefore, patient education is not in the front of their minds. You may not be able to change this, but there are a couple of tricks you may wish to try.

Place a poster about your program in the doctor's waiting room or examining room. Have patients tear off tags with the phone number for more information. This way, the doctor does not have to do anything, yet the patient understands that the doctor approves of the program. In addition, the poster acts as a stimulus for the patient to ask the doctor for more information or reminds the doctor about the program. Be sure to institute a system to replace these posters regularly.

A second method of enlisting help with recruitment from a doctor or other health professional is to get permission to place a brightly colored sign-up sheet in the professional's waiting room. The front of the sheet should say something like "I am interested in learning more about diabetes education," and this should be followed by spaces for names, addresses, and phone numbers. The other side of the sheet should be preaddressed and pre-stamped. Ask the office receptionist to take down the sheet and mail it to you every 2 weeks or when the sheet is full, whichever occurs first. In turn, you send him or her a new sheet. This takes all the responsibility away from the doctor and gets you the information you need. By the way, thank-you notes and occasional small gifts go a long way toward getting the cooperation of over-worked and often underappreciated office staff.

A third method of getting doctor referrals is to make up special prescription pads (small printers can do this inexpensively). The doctor then prescribes patient education in much the same way he or she would prescribe medication. Some programs require a doctor's signature before people can attend. If this is the case, include a place on the physician referral (permission) form where the doctor can request material about the program for his or her office (see Figure 5.1).

Many physicians have told us that they do not refer because there are so many programs and so many places to refer that they cannot remember them all. One solution is one-stop shopping. All the physician has to do is say, "I want you to learn more about _____. Please go and see Mary Smith and she will suggest ways you can do this." It is then Mary Smith's job to talk with patients in person, by phone, or via e-mail. She can suggest the various alternatives.

Now that automated medical records are becoming more common, these can be used for recruitment. First generate a list of all the patients with a specific target condition and ask the physician to sort this list, then give the list to the patients' physicians and ask each physician to cross off anyone who should not be invited to the program. Letters can then be sent to everyone remaining on the list, inviting them to the program. Such letters will be more powerful if the patient's personal physician signs them.

Self-Management Study
Stanford University School of Medicine
Department of Medicine

Please return to:

Stanford Patient Education Research Center
1000 Welch Road, Suite 204
Palo Alto, California 94304
(415) 723-7935
(415) 723-9656 FAX

Patient's Name: _____

Address: _____

DIAGNOSIS: My patient has one or more of the following diseases and is age 40 or over. He/she does not have compromised mentation nor has he/she received radiation or chemotherapy for cancer within the past year.

PLEASE CHECK ALL DIAGNOSES THAT APPLY:

☐ Asthma

☐ Chronic bronchitis

☐ Emphysema/COPD

☐ Other chronic lung disease

   *Specify type:*_____

☐ Coronary artery disease

   with angina or congestive

   heart failure

☐ Completed cerebrovascular accident **with**
   neurological handicap and normal mentation

☐ Osteoarthritis

☐ Rheumatoid arthritis

☐ Other rheumatic disease

   *Specify type:*_____

☐ Other chronic disease

   *Specify type:*_____

_____   _____
      DATE   SIGNATURE OF PHYSICIAN

                  _____
                  PRINT name of physician

I am interested in referring patients to your study. Please send me:
☐ **Brochures**   #_____
☐ **Exam room posters** #_____
☐ **Prescription pads** #_____
My address is:

Figure 5.1. Sample Physician Referral Form for a Patient Education Program

A final way to gain the support of physicians is to allow them to see the program and be sure that they receive patient feedback. You might invite different physicians to be on a panel during the program. This allows them to "see" the program while being part of it. Also, ask patients to tell their doctors about the program. In one program we know of, participants are urged to write letters to their doctors about the program. Satisfied patients are a powerful tool for getting physician buy-in.

Some health plans, hospitals, or clinics have newsletters in which you can advertise your program. Because it is affiliated with a respected source, your program becomes acceptable. When using newsletters to advertise, be very sure your program's telephone number is published. Telling people about your program does no good if they do not know how to contact you.

Sometimes doctors fear that the education program will somehow interfere with their treatment or chase patients into the hands of other practitioners. To overcome this fear, first assure the doctors that you will always refer their patients back to them—and be sure to do so. Second, you might offer to hold the program after hours in the doctor's waiting room. This solves your space problem and ensures that a specific doctor is associated with that session of the program.

Within your program, and in your dealings with the public, be very sure to teach that doctors are not the enemy. Too often, there is a subtle or not-so-subtle implication that patients must be on the defensive with doctors. Avoid this at all costs. Also, do not play favorites. Even though you may like one doctor better than another, *always* support the patient's choice of doctor. If there are medical questions, suggest that the patient ask his or her doctor. If a patient is unhappy with the doctor, urge a patient-doctor discussion. A doctor once said that doctors will get off their pedestals when patients get off their knees. Our job is to help patients stand, not to knock doctors off their pedestals.

One final note: Unless your program is well-known and established, you will probably not get many of your referrals from physicians. Rather, you must market directly to the public. The following sections should be helpful.

☒ MARKETING TO THE PUBLIC

Making Your Program Attractive

Much of the problem in recruiting patients may be that your program is not attractive. Some of the common problems are the program's name, cost, time, place, and length.

Name

The name of your program is very important. "Self-Help for the Elderly" forces participants to admit they are old before enrolling. "Growing Younger and Healthier" might be a better title. Hypertension is a symptomless disease, so there may be little motivation on the part of many patients to attend a program. On the other hand, chronic obstructive pulmonary disease (COPD) has painful symptoms; therefore, it might be easier to recruit for "COPD Better Breathers" programs. Sometimes, programs with more than one focus can help. Because a large percentage of older people have arthritis, you might reach more elderly hypertensives with an arthritis and high blood pressure program than with just a high blood pressure program. One way to choose a name while also resolving some of the other issues discussed in this section is to use focus groups. You will find details about this technique in Chapter 1.

Sometimes programs have names that are not well understood by patients. For example, "Chronic Disease Self-Management" is not clear, because many people do not understand either *chronic disease* or *self-management.* A better name might be "Living a Healthy Life With Long-Term Conditions." Also, people sometimes respond better to the word *workshop* than they do

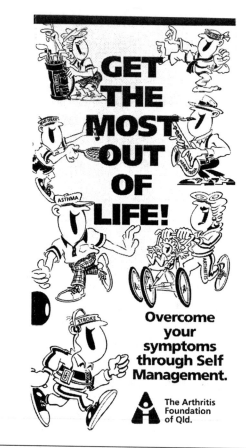

Figure 5.2. Example of Program Publicity Material

SOURCE: The Arthritis Foundation of Queensland.

to *course* or *program*. Figure 5.2 illustrates publicity for a chronic disease program.

Some final hints about naming programs:

- Don't be too cute. Illness is a serious matter, especially to the ill. Treating it frivolously often causes anger.

- Keep the name simple. No one wants to deal with a 14-word name.

- Make the name descriptive. The name is what initially attracts people. "Asthma Self-Management," "Avoiding Heart Attacks," "How to Talk With Your Doctor," and "Preparing for Labor" are all good, clear, descriptive titles. "Aches and Pains" is cute, but it is not very descriptive.

Cost

There is a widely held belief among health professionals and others that if people pay for something, they value it more. Although this may be true, we have little evidence to suggest that payment makes much difference in terms of behavior change or health status outcome. In fact, if payment were directly linked to outcome, the United States would have the healthiest population in the world! The point here is that you do not have to charge money to make patients appreciate your program. On the other hand, payment may influence attendance or commitment. For example, some weight-loss programs charge a high fee and then offer rebates for prespecified weight loss and weight-loss maintenance. It is true that people who prepay usually show up. However, the same results can be accomplished by having people preregister, especially if the preregistration requires filling out a written form. In our evaluation studies, we have found that when people fill out a questionnaire before attending the first class, the no-show rate is less than 10%.

You may need to charge to cover the expenses of the program. Usually, the lower or more minimal the fee, the better. This makes your program accessible to everyone. If you must charge more than a minimal fee, you might try a sliding scale. Your application can state that the program costs $25 but that considerations will be made for those with limited income. Then, as part of the application, have participants check one of the following:

Enclosed is $25.00.

I can afford only $_____; enclosed is $_____.

Please consider me for a fee waiver _____.

If the fee is reasonable, people usually do not take advantage of this offer. In our experience with an arthritis patient education program (the Arthritis Self-Help Course), most people pay the full fee, and very few request a complete scholarship. When we have charged $15 to $20, less than 5% of more than 1,000 patients have asked for fee waivers. All the rest have paid the full fee. When the cost of the course is raised to $30 to $40, attendance is affected. Today, with the spread of health maintenance organizations and other prepaid plans, patient education is often budgeted as part of ongoing patient services. If this is not true in your area, part of your job is to advocate for formal patient education to be a part of ongoing budgeted services. Often, some of the course expenses can be paid for from other sources. For more information on this, see the section on using community resources later in this chapter.

A note about requesting funding: Start with the premise that patient education is no longer a nice extra. Rather, if you are offering evidence-based programs, patient education is a proven form of treatment that enhances health status or slows decline. In addition, it is often cost-effective. To neglect to offer patients this treatment is to provide suboptimal care. The Center for the Advancement of Health publishes extensive annotated bibliographies and newsletters of patient education studies that you can use to bolster your funding requests.[1]

Time

It seems obvious that you should hold your program at a convenient time for the clients. Saturday may be a sports day for you but a very lonely day for the elderly. We have held about 30% of our programs on Saturday mornings. Also, take a look at your competition. Do not hold your hypertension program during the Olympics or on church bingo nights. However, it might be successful if you hold it at the bingo hall half an hour before bingo begins. You may even consider offering more than one program on different days, at different times, in order to reach more people.

You should also consider the length of your program. Once programs get to be longer than 5 to 7 weeks, completion is a problem. Although 2 hours a week for 5 or 6 weeks may be convenient for city dwellers, people in rural areas who must travel long distances may find it more convenient to attend two half-day sessions.

Place

People are funny. Some places are all right to go to and others are not. This has nothing to do with safety. If you want to reach an ethnic population, you might have more success holding the program in a community setting rather than in a hospital, but be careful: A place that looks just fine to you, such as a new Asian youth activity center, may be uncomfortable for some participants, such as older Asians. Some Catholics may not be willing to go to a Protestant church for a program, and vice versa, whereas others will. Also, some people may be willing to cross town for a program, but won't cross the railroad tracks. People have set ranges, and your program must be given within the range of your audience. Your task is to find out what that range is, perhaps through your needs assessment or in a focus group.

Of course, sites must be safe and accessible. Things to consider are stairs, other impediments to the physically challenged, parking, public transportation, walking distance, lighting, comfort of chairs, accessibility of toilets, and facilities for making coffee and tea. If you are teaching wellness or prevention, hospitals may not be the best places because, in people's minds, that is where sick people go. Hospitals have a negative image for some people. They are also full of things they perceive as strange and frightening, and they have peculiar smells. In addition, parking and access for the general public may require a lot of walking. For this reason, try to hold your course on neutral ground. Shopping malls, pubs, hotels, town halls, senior centers, and libraries usually meet this criterion. They are accessible and acceptable to a wide spectrum of the population (see the section on using community resources later in this chapter).

Using the Media

So you have done everything right, and still no one comes. It may be that no one knew about your program. Good advertising is done in a number of ways. The local media, radio and newspapers, are excellent but are also unpredictable if you rely solely on public service announcements. The problem is that you never know when your announcement will be published or broadcast. Nevertheless, you should send press releases to all your local media. These should be short and ready to use (see Figures 5.3 and 5.4 for some examples). Unfortunately, paid advertising is very expensive. However, for something really important, this may be the way to go. Again, it is important to know the audience. You would not want to advertise a prenatal program for teens on an all-news radio station.

Sometimes when you are starting a new program or have a new angle on an old program, you can get a newspaper to do a feature story. If this happens, be sure that the story includes information on how you can be reached. The best story in the world is useless if your address or phone number is not included. On radio, the equivalent of a feature story is a short interview or, better still, a segment on a talk show. Again, it is important that you somehow get in the information on how to contact you. In fact, on radio, this should be done several times, because listeners may not get all the information the first time it is given.

Stanford Patient Education Research Center

Stanford University School of Medicine
Department of Medicine

1000 Welch Road. Suite 204
Palo Alto. California 94304
(650) 723-7935
(650) 723-9656 FAX

CALENDAR ANNOUNCEMENT

May, 2000

Contact: **Maria Hernández**
                (650) 723-7935

SELF-MANAGEMENT PROGRAM

FOR HEART CONDITIONS, LUNG CONDITIONS, ARTHRITIS

Fatigue, frustration, pain, limitations? If so, this Self-Management Course has been designed just for you. The course, developed by the Stanford University School of Medicine's Patient Education Research Center, teaches people 40 and over to cope with the symptoms and frustrations of living with a chronic condition. The course is offered at various locations in San Francisco, San Mateo, Santa Clara and Alameda counties. **Classes will begin in July, 2000.** Because it is a research project, there is no charge. Enrollment is limited and pre-registration is required through Stanford. For more information and registration, contact the Stanford Patient Education Research Center at **1-800-366-2624.**

Figure 5.3. Sample Announcement of a Patient Education Program

Aside from the large mass media, all communities have a number of club, church, and other newsletters. Putting your announcement in those targeted to your audience can be both effective and inexpensive. The problem with these is that they usually have a long lead time. Thus if you want something published the first of January, it may have to be in by early November.

Stanford Patient Education Research Center

Stanford University School of Medicine
Department of Medicine

1000 Welch Road. Suite 204
Palo Alto. California 94304
(650) 723-7935
(650) 723-9656 FAX

NEWS RELEASE
July, 2000

Living Well With Chronic Conditions Workshop

Are you sick and tired of your chronic health problem? If so, you are invited to take part in the Living Well With Chronic Conditions Workshop sponsored by the Stanford Patient Education Research Center. In the six-week workshop, you will learn about symptom management, medication "how to's", working with your doctor, dealing with negative emotions, and the latest in exercise. In addition, we will help you design and carry out your own self-management program.

Courses are offered at many sites throughout the Bay Area starting in September, 2000. Pre-registration is required and enrollment is limited. Anyone with chronic health conditions, their spouses and friends, are welcome. For more information and registration, call the Stanford Patient Education Research Center toll free at **1-800-366-2624**.

Figure 5.4. Sample News Release for a Patient Education Program

Sometimes correspondence sent by fax or e-mail receives more attention than that sent by conventional mail. It is useful to keep a file of all media sources, contact persons, and lead times.

Flyers can also be effective if well placed. I have found that good places for flyers are on the cash registers at local pharmacies, in doctors' waiting rooms, at public libraries, in beauty and barber shops, and in local markets and shops. Sometimes, as in the case of an AIDS education program, it is helpful to hand out flyers on the street. Flyers can also be distributed by such organizations as Meals on Wheels. Sometimes, you have to be really creative. If you are trying to reach a young audience, try putting flyers in fitness centers. Families with young children are often found in toy stores and fast-food restaurants—advertise in those places. If you are trying to reach older populations, you might include a flyer in the program of the Sunday afternoon armchair travel program. Don't forget the Internet—many health organizations have Web sites. List your programs on your own Web site and ask community groups to link to your site. Of course, return the favor by providing links to their sites.

One final and excellent source of publicity is word of mouth. To use this, let past participants know about future programs. Ask them to post flyers in places that they frequent and also to tell their friends. You might even send past participants postcards that their friends can send in for more information. We have found this to be one of the very best sources of publicity.

Once you have gone through all the trouble of publicizing in many places, it is nice to know what is effective. The easiest way of doing this is by having a place on your application where people can write in where they found out about your program. In this way, you can track your publicity and keep using those sources that are effective while eliminating those that are not. Also be sure to ask anyone calling for information how he or she found out about your program.

Community Talks: Reaching the Hard to Reach

One of the biggest problems for many patient educators is reaching patients who are hard to reach. Often, we consider those people who are not like ourselves or like our regular clients to be hard to reach. In English-speaking countries, most health care professionals speak English as their primary language; therefore, the hard to reach might be defined as those whose primary language is not English. The poor and elderly are other groups that are usually defined as hard to reach. As if to prove that the definition of who is hard to reach is a matter of perception, some health educators from Puerto Rico have told us that they have had difficulty accessing members of the English-speaking community.

In trying to identify ways to reach these groups, a good place to start is by looking at who is reaching them. Where and to whom do they go for information and service? By this, we mean, where do they buy their food and clothing, and where are their social and sports activities? Why are these services successful when yours are not? At the same time, examine what happens when the hard to reach enter your health care system. Are there people who speak their language and understand their customs? Are your services located in a convenient place? Are people treated courteously? The ultimate question to ask yourself is, If I were them, would I use our services?

In planning your program, you also want to ask yourself whether you really want to reach them. This sounds harsh, but it is important to consider *before* beginning your outreach efforts. Really wanting to reach them means being willing and able to commit the resources—the staff, time, and money—to develop and maintain services in those communities. If you do not make efforts to provide ongoing funding or if you pull out of a community too fast without helping them develop resources and maintain the program, bad feelings, tension, and distrust are likely to result. This makes it difficult for anyone to work in that community in the future. Therefore, establishing and maintaining good community relations are also important.

The primary rule in trying to reach the hard to reach is to go to them. Do not expect them to come to you. This includes your telephone system. If at all possible, have a dedicated line that is always answered in the language of the population you are trying to reach. For more information on working competently with persons from diverse cultures, see Chapter 6.

✪ USING COMMUNITY RESOURCES

Every community has resources. Finding them is the problem. Sometimes, the problem is not really finding them but rather seeing what is before your eyes. For example, every community has hotels, bars, and restaurants. However, we seldom think of these as sites for patient education. In fact, many of these establishments spend a great deal of their time nearly empty. Thus you might be able to use a bar or a restaurant for a morning class. These sites might be especially attractive if you are trying to reach men. Hotel swimming pools are used heavily in the early mornings and in the evenings. However, between those times, they might be used for a water exercise class. Similarly, doctors all have empty waiting rooms when patients are not being seen; these might be used for evening classes.

Service clubs are also common in most communities. Lions, Rotary, and Apex are all groups that you can call upon for help. One of the missions of these groups is community service, and with a little creative thinking, you can help them fulfill their mission. Members of these organizations can be recruited to get people to courses or to give public lectures. Also, most communities have a variety of youth groups, such as Scouts and Guides. Members of these organizations can be trained as peer counselors or as baby-sitters for handicapped children or adults. They are also experts at distributing flyers or announcements. As a special project, they might even design some of your patient education materials. Give them a chance to do their daily good turn. Organizations such as police and firefighter groups, unions, and farm clubs can also be most helpful.

In large communities, it is often difficult to get access to the media. However, just the opposite is sometimes true in smaller towns. Newspapers and radio stations need material. You may arrange to do a weekly newspaper column or to broadcast a stress management program twice weekly over the radio. You will never find out what you can get if you do not ask.

Most merchants are constantly asked for things. Try asking for something different. For example, in a big city, ask a major department store to help you advertise an event. In turn, you can go through the store and help the store's marketing people identify products that they can feature for pregnant women, the elderly, the handicapped, and so on. Thus you are helping them to increase their customer base.

In places that are very hot, cold, or wet, walking and other outdoor exercises are sometimes a problem. Most of these same communities also have enclosed areas, such as malls, office buildings, airports, or markets, that can be used for walking programs in the hours before opening. In large cities, airports have miles of climate-controlled corridors that are good for walking. One elderly group walks inside a shopping mall two mornings a week from 8:00 a.m. to 9:00 a.m. and then has coffee and a health lecture in the mall coffee shop. Because there are few people in the mall before the shops open at 9:00 a.m., the owner is pleased to get the extra business. Walking tracks can be marked out with colored tape: Once around the mall equals a quarter mile, or two flights of stairs equal a 100-foot elevation gain.

You can find skilled personnel in much the same way you find sites for your program. Many communities have volunteer bureaus. If you have special needs, ask. Many people would volunteer if they did not have to lick envelopes or be president of something. If there are no volunteer bureaus, make your needs known through church bulletins or local newspapers. You never know what will happen. Students are another wonderful source of assistance. Although health professional students are an obvious source of help, think more broadly. For example, information technology students might help you create and maintain a Web site.

All of the above is fine and good, but what if what you really need is money? The place to start is near home. It is important to make clear to your organization that patient education is not merely a nice add-on service. It is an integral part of patient care.

As such, it must be budgeted for in much the same way as nursing services. Good basic patient education programs usually cost one-quarter to one-half of 1% of an organization's total budget. This basic budget can be supplemented by donations from service clubs and churches and by grants from foundations and merchants. Most of these organizations have planned giving programs, so they will not instantly hand over cash. However, if you understand their programs and how to ask for money through their channels, you may well get what you need.

Beyond local organizations, look to government groups: local, state, or national. Again, there are all kinds of rules and regulations. However, if you are willing to play the game and have a good product, you may well get the funding you need. In dealing with bureaucracies, remember to play by the rules: Dot all the i's and cross all the t's. Be sure that the government officials who will fund your request understand your program and are sold on it. After all, they will be the ones to present it to the people higher up. Finally, have enough time. You probably cannot find the funds you need in a week. However, any program that is worth doing today is probably still worth doing in 6 months.

No matter what you are asking for, one of the best ways to get it is by asking the person or organization you are approaching about how to get what you want, the principle being that people usually want to be helpful. For example, if you want the local radio station to air a stress management series, ask the station manager what you would need to do to get such a series on the air. He or she will then outline a number of things for you to do. Listen carefully and write these down. Then, do just what he or she says. If you do this, it will be very difficult for the manager to keep your series off the air. When people tell you how to do something and you follow through, they have almost committed themselves to do it.

In short, all communities have resources. Your job is to recognize, find, and, most important, use them effectively.

◘ **NOTE**

1. The Center for the Advancement of Health has developed indexed bibliographies on self-management of asthma, diabetes, cardiovascular disease (CVD), low back pain, and alcohol misuses. They also have newsletters and are constantly developing new directories of evidence-based behavioral interventions. Best of all, most materials are free. To obtain any of these, contact the Center for the Advancement of Health, 2000 Florida Avenue, NW, Suite 210, Washington, DC 20009; fax (202) 387-2857; phone (202) 387-3829; Web site http://www.cfah.org.

6

Working Cross-Culturally

Virginia M. González
Kate Lorig

W orking cross-culturally can be challenging to even the most experienced health professional; it can also be some of the most interesting and rewarding work you will ever do. The way you approach the challenge will determine the success of your efforts. For example, if you choose to develop an educational program that respects and incorporates the cultural beliefs and practices of a group, you are more likely to be successful than if you simply translate or transplant an existing program from one group to another without making any adaptations.

In this chapter, we discuss some practical guidelines to help you work more effectively and comfortably with diverse cultural groups and to develop culturally appropriate patient education programs. We have also included a list of additional references at the end of this chapter that provide more specific and in-depth information on this topic. Before we do that, however, it is important to explain what is meant by key concepts such as *culture, cultural identity,* and *ethnic identity* and how these contribute to diversity.

¤ UNDERSTANDING CULTURAL DIVERSITY

Culture is a shared set of beliefs, assumptions, values, and practices; it determines how we interpret and interact with the world and structures our behavior and attitudes throughout our lives. An individual's or group's culture strongly determines the way in which the individual or group defines health and illness. For example, in some cultural groups, health and illness are defined by the balance or imbalance of spiritual or supernatural forces rather than by biological, behavioral, or environmental factors alone. An appreciation and respect for these different beliefs and practices, as well as an understanding of how they differ from your own, will greatly enhance your ability to work with different cultural groups. This, in turn, will increase the effectiveness of your programs.

In planning and implementing patient education programs, it is important to realize that the individuals or groups you are targeting may actually have more than one cultural identity. Such variation in cultural identities within groups reflects the influence of several factors and individuals' responses to their experience with these factors:

- Historical, socioeconomic, and political experiences in the homeland and new country
- Education
- Family and peer influence
- Native or primary language

- Religion
- Age at time of immigration
- Place of residence and length of time in the new country
- Citizenship status
- Whether the individual lives in an integrated community

A person's cultural identity is dynamic, changing as a result of contact with different groups. This process of change, or acculturation, occurs naturally over time. It refers to the acquisition of a new cultural identity but does not preclude retention of the old; a person may become bicultural, identifying with two different cultures (the old and new). Each individual has his or her own process of integrating the new culture with the old. Cultural diversity is the result of this interaction between different cultures. Individuals and groups create new cultural identities that are often a synthesis of separate and disparate cultures. For example, many immigrant groups have chosen to maintain the practices of their cultural heritage (i.e., their language, religion, and traditions) while also acquiring, to varying degrees and in different ways, some of the values, practices, and language of the new culture in order to function in the larger society.

The extreme form of acculturation is assimilation, in which the individual or group completely incorporates the new culture. Gradually, the values, practices, or traditions of the native culture, particularly those that do not conform to the standards of the new group, are lost or given up and replaced by those of the new group.

Understanding that diversity exists within and between cultures will help you avoid the tendency to form cultural stereotypes about a group with which you have had limited experience. One of the biggest mistakes you can make as a patient educator is to base your actions on inaccurate assumptions, misconceptions, oversimplifications, or generalizations about a patient's culture. By doing so, you might create a program or act in a way that is at best inappropriate and at worst offensive to the people you are trying to serve.

With this in mind, let's look at how to learn more about the cultural diversity of your patient population.

¤ WHERE TO START

If you are not sure which cultural groups you want to serve, start by gathering some specific information about your general patient population. For example, what are the demographic characteristics of the population? This includes information about age, sex, education, marital status, place of birth, ethnic origin, language spoken, type of health problems, and services used. Answers to these questions can help you better define your target groups, as well as learn something about their cultural identities and levels of acculturation. It can be misleading, however, to rely solely on demographic information in this process, especially if the questions or forms used to collect this information are not very specific. For example, in answering a question about ethnic origin, both Chinese and Japanese persons would check the category *Asian*; however, if asked to be specific, they would probably prefer to respond with *Chinese* or *Japanese*, respectively. Therefore, although ethnic categories can help identify groups, they do not always provide enough information. One's ethnicity is not necessarily the same as one's culture. People from countries such as China, India, and the Philippines and from geographic regions such as Latin America might indicate the same ethnicity (e.g., Chinese, Indian, Filipino, or Hispanic/ Latino) but actually belong to distinct cultural or language groups. Therefore, if your program needs to be this specific, you may need to identify languages spoken and the specific traditions in addition to ethnicity.

There are also other distinctions you can make to learn more about your population. For example, if you have identified a large Spanish-speaking population for whom you would like to develop a program, try to find out if the individuals involved are from the same country or from different regions of Latin America. This is important to know because, although people from different regions may all speak Spanish, they may hold some very different health beliefs and be accustomed to different health practices. Also, depending on their level of acculturation, they may be monolingual or bilingual and have different language preferences. Often, older adults will prefer using their native language, whereas teenagers might be more comfortable communicating in English. Also, some may prefer to speak their native language but read and write English. All of this information is relevant and important to consider when developing educational programs and materials for diverse groups.

Therefore, when you are attempting to determine the level of acculturation with respect to the culture you wish to serve, it is helpful to ask questions about language preferences when speaking, reading, and writing, as well as about length of time in the country. Some acculturation scales that were developed for use with different ethnic groups in the United States can be modified to help you with this task.

Another consideration to help you identify cultural groups is whether patients have common experiences. For example, although both World War II and Vietnam War veterans fought and survived a war, they had very different specific experiences. They represent two distinct cultural groups and may require very different types of educational programs or services.

After you have identified your target groups, you can start gathering more specific information about the cultures. (Table 6.1 presents a list of some of the questions you should consider in your search.) An easy and more personal approach to gathering this information is to ask several individuals from the group. For example, you might ask several patients through informal conversations or semistructured interviews. You might also talk with their family members. The bits of information gathered from each patient should help you form a better understanding of some of their cultural beliefs and practices. At the same time, you can reciprocate by sharing with them some of your beliefs and practices. Such exchange promotes the cross-cultural understanding of both provider and patient and helps to build trust and rapport; these are important for the success of your future efforts.

There are also more formal ways of gathering this information from your patient population. These include the use of focus groups and questionnaires. These techniques are discussed in more detail in Chapter 1.

You can also gather information at the library by reading different types of literature about the population to be served. For example, you may want to review historical documents or tapes about the group; these may give you a greater understanding and appreciation for their current circumstances. Also, try to read appropriate medical or public health literature that describes the results of other programs or studies with this population. Behavioral and social science literature, especially ethnic studies or anthropological materials, may provide a general understanding of different cultural beliefs and practices. Finally, read the local newspapers, listen to the radio, or watch television, especially any ethnic newspapers or programming targeting the groups you are interested in serving. (If you have never seen ethnic newspapers, magazines, or programs in your local area or region, this does not mean they do not exist. You may have to hunt to find them. Start by asking your patients; they can be your guides and interpreters, if necessary.) These can help you to gain some insight into the community's problems and concerns and also help you identify people, places, and events to consider later in the development and implementation of your program or

TABLE 6.1 Questions to Consider in Gathering Information on a Target Group's Culture

What name or names do individuals use to define their cultural or ethnic identity (e.g., *German, Hispanic, Mexican, Polish, Latino*)?

What is the significance of each name?

What are some major differences between or within cultural groups, particularly across generational, educational, socioeconomic, and geographic lines?

What are the different education and/or literacy levels within groups? Are individuals literate/illiterate in their own language, English, or both?

How many and which languages or dialects are spoken? Is there a common language understood by all? Is there a written language?

What type of medical care did group members have in their native country?

How is medical care used by these different groups?

What are the expectations for doctors, nurses, and other health professionals?

What are the values of the group or groups you wish to serve?

What are some of the more common health beliefs and practices of the various members of different groups?

What are the predominant family structures in the group you wish to serve (hierarchical, patriarchal, two-parent household, single-parent household, female-headed household, extended, nuclear)?

What are some of the traditional roles of different family members, particularly where health is concerned?

Who are the formal and informal leaders in the community, and what role do they play with regard to health, health care, and education?

What are the formal and informal channels of communication used by your target group?

What are group members' general beliefs about the cause, prevention, diagnosis, and treatment of different diseases or health problems?

What are group members' specific beliefs about the health problem that you are trying to address?

services. A reference librarian may also be able to suggest other sources of information.

A third way to gather information is to talk with other people who know something about the community you wish to serve. These may be other professionals working in and with the same community or may be your friends, colleagues, or coworkers. They can provide yet another perspective about the culture; however, they will be able to report only their own experiences. Also, their experiences may not be representative of those of the patients you are trying to access, or they may not feel qualified to comment. After all, most of us would feel uncomfortable if asked to describe our own culture.

Finally, try visiting the communities in which your patients live. Good community reconnaissance can give you valuable information on how to build a program. Visits should be made at different times of the day on weekdays and weekends so that you can get a good picture of what is happening in the community; this also allows you to be seen. The more time you spend there, the more likely it is that you will become recognized by members of that community.

The best approach in gathering information about your target group is to employ a variety of these methods. In this way, your sources of information will be varied and, it is hoped, less likely to present you with false stereotypes.

✿ HOW DO I CREATE A CULTURALLY APPROPRIATE PROGRAM?

Creating a culturally appropriate program is no different than creating any other patient education program. You start out with a needs assessment (see Chapter 1), write your objectives (see Chapter 4), and then design a program (see Chapter 4). The only difference is that you take into account and incorporate the appropriate cultural information you learned earlier about the target group. One change in your program might be something as simple as offering the program in a community setting instead of at the hospital or clinic. Or you might have to make more creative changes in the content and process of the program so that it is more relevant. For example, if a group's diet emphasizes certain foods, such as rice and noodles, as staples, then content related to nutrition, making dietary changes, or both may need to emphasize these foods rather than potatoes and bread. Also, methods of instruction may need to be modified. For example, if there are varying levels of literacy within the group, you may need to rely on audio- or videotapes rather than written materials for instruction. If the group has definite beliefs about causes of and treatments for certain health problems, then these should be integrated into the teaching.

This is the time to work collaboratively with other people who are bicultural and able to help you make the necessary changes. Ideally, these people should feel very comfortable in both the culture you wish to reach and the majority culture. Although it would also be nice if they have some professional training or expertise in the health field, this is not always possible or realistic. It is important, however, that you, the community, and, it is hoped, your organization trust their cultural expertise. The individuals you identify and choose to work with in the development and implementation of your program must have the trust and respect of the community to ensure the program's credibility and success. One way to gain trust and ensure credibility is to hire individuals from the community to assist with various tasks during different phases of the program's development and implementation.

The success of your program is determined not only by its cultural relevance and the community's acceptance but by your organization's commitment to serving a culturally diverse population. This commitment to promote cultural diversity is evidenced in how the organization (a) allocates its resources to ensure that quality care and services are both accessible and responsive to the needs of all patients and (b) works to develop collaborative relationships (formal and informal) with different agencies in the ethnic communities it serves. For example, the organization should be committed to recruiting and employing not only ancillary staff from the community but professional staff who can provide clinically, culturally, and linguistically proficient services. Also, your organization might contract services with businesses in that community and endorse or cosponsor community events.

If your organization is not able to make such commitments, it is unlikely that your program will be long lived. Therefore, it is important to investigate how and where you might institutionalize your program if it is successful during your planning process. Otherwise, the patients and community may become angry and less willing to work with you or your organization in the future. Lack of commitment and follow-through in the community can adversely affect your reputation and that of your organization.

¤ STRATEGIES FOR ADAPTING PROGRAM CONTENT AND PROCESS

Adapting a program's content and process for different cultures involves more than just translating the information. It also involves the following:

- Changing the actual health information into different, more specific, or more relevant terminology
- Creating new descriptions or explanations that fit better with different people's understanding of key concepts
- Incorporating a group's cultural beliefs and practices into the program content and process

With the help of others, such as an advisory group made up of representatives of the community you wish to serve and/or bilingual, bicultural consultants, review the different sources of information you gathered to identify the culture-specific beliefs and practices about the problem you will address. Use this information to decide how and where to focus the health education efforts. For example, are you interested in providing information to correct certain myths or misconceptions about health, are you attempting to change people's health behaviors, or are you trying to identify and modify some of the environmental factors or barriers that affect either or both health and access to health care? Let us examine each of these strategies more closely.

Dispelling Health Misconceptions and Myths

Misconceptions and myths about health, disease, or illness are usually based on incorrect or incomplete information. Therefore, one educational strategy might be to correct these misconceptions by helping people reinterpret what they know about the health problem. You can do this by providing more accurate or less confusing explanations about a health problem or by providing new experiences for people to try, helping them reinterpret their understanding of a disease. For example, some individuals and groups believe that arthritis is a fatal disease. This belief is usually based on their own experiences of having seen or known people who suffered greatly with arthritis. They lack complete information about what arthritis is, the types of arthritis, and the importance of treatment to prevent serious problems or complications (e.g., death). If this is the case, your educational efforts might focus on providing more information about the different types of arthritis and appropriate treatments. As a general rule, when providing this new information, you should try to limit the use of technical jargon. If you must use technical words, try to explain or define them in lay terms. Also, whenever possible, use visual aids and culturally relevant analogies to help people understand concepts that are complex, abstract, or totally foreign. Another approach might be to help people with arthritis reinterpret what is happening with their disease when they experience changes related to a particular treatment. For example, explain what a specific medication or treatment is doing for them. How is it changing the symptoms they had before? How are they feeling now as a result of the treatment? In this case, the actual experience of the treatment may help to dispel their misconceptions about the disease.

Other misconceptions are formed when people misinterpret the words or messages used to inform them about a disease. For example, some of the misconceptions people have about the transmission of the AIDS virus come from misinterpretations of vague phrases, such as *bodily fluids,* that were used in early educational campaigns. This vagueness led many people to believe that the virus could be transmitted easily through contact with any or all of the body's fluids, including saliva, perspiration, and tears, which is not the case.

Changing Behavior

Sometimes it is easier to change people's behavior by teaching them new skills than it is to try to change health beliefs and values. People's beliefs and values are usually integral parts of a whole system of understanding (i.e., culture) and are strongly held. Even if the beliefs and values of a group's members seem harmful or unhealthy to you, individuals are not likely to change because you point out what is wrong with those beliefs. In fact, doing that would not only be insensitive but would alienate group members. Rather, it is best to try to change behaviors by incorporating, not changing, existing beliefs and values.

For example, among some ethnic groups there is strong belief in the hot-cold theory of disease. The terms *hot* and *cold* in this context do not refer to temperature but rather to four bodily fluids (sometimes called *humors*) that have certain designations. For example, blood is considered to be hot and wet, yellow bile is hot and dry, phlegm is cold and wet, and black bile is cold and dry. When all these are balanced, the body is healthy; any imbalance causes illness or disease. If a disease is considered hot and wet, the appropriate treatment would have to be the opposite, cold and dry. Therefore, rather than trying to change such an ingrained belief, find out from your patient exactly what foods or medications are considered acceptable treatments for a particular health problem and integrate these into the activities designed to change behaviors. This approach was used by a nutrition educator working with a group of elderly people with type 2 diabetes who believed diabetes was a "hot" disease. In helping them learn how to modify their diets to control the diabetes, she identified foods not only by their nutrients but also by their functions. Therefore, she was able to emphasize those ethnic foods the elders considered "cold" when teaching them how to plan their meals. Because she incorporated their belief rather than trying to change it, these elderly were more compliant and better able to control their diabetes through diet.

When culturally adapting activities that encourage behavior change, integrate not only those beliefs or practices specific to health but also others, such as those around food, religion or spirituality, family, music, and exercise. Depending on the cultural group, many of these may be related to perceptions about health as well as health practices.

Changing the Organizational Environment

Patient educators need to work not only with patients to change behaviors but with health care organizations to identify and change environmental factors that affect their patients' ability to access appropriate services. In this role, the educator becomes a patient advocate and spokesperson, identifying and suggesting ways in which organization administrators might begin to revise policies and procedures so as to value and promote diversity across the board. If organizations can do this in a meaningful way, they may find that more costly services, such as emergency and urgent care, are reduced.

Program Tips

The following are some specific tips to help you begin adapting program content and process for different cultural groups.

1. *Use a multilevel approach.* Making a program more culturally appropriate often means choosing different strategies to tackle different levels of the problem. In this way, the changes achieved are relevant to the individual's health as well as to other aspects of the individual's life (e.g., social, economic conditions, physical environment). For example, a diabetes education program might focus on teaching patients how to make necessary changes in diet and eating habits while also working with the family to help support these changes and local community markets to label or identify healthful food products more efficiently for people with diabetes.

2. *Do more than translate materials.* Literal translations often result in a product that is inappropriate or even absurd to the target group. It is much better to create new materials from scratch on the basis of the information you have gathered. These can then be pilot tested on focus groups, who help you to refine the materials. If you need to rely on translated materials, refer to the section on methods of translation later in this chapter.

3. *Incorporate different types of music, art, drama, or dance into your patient education activities.* For example, one health department organized a senior theater group whose musical performances demonstrated common medication problems and how seniors might avoid them. The actors were all seniors who represented the ethnic diversity of the community. These plays were given at senior centers and senior housing projects.

4. *Try to personalize the delivery of your program.* Many cultural groups prefer the personal, one-on-one or small-group approach. Personalizing can be as simple as training staff and volunteers to be warm and friendly with community people, rather than aloof and businesslike. It might also include sending invitations or personalized letters to the people you want to attend, followed up with phone calls as reminders, or encouraging people to call each other during the week as part of the program. Finally, consider a community-based site such as a church or community center rather than the hospital or clinic for the program.

5. *Include different family members as much as possible in the delivery and dissemination of patient education programs.* For example, if elders are the primary source of health advice, train them first to educate others. If you are offering classes, invite family members and significant others to attend. Arrange for transportation and child care as needed. When addressing delicate issues such as men's or women's health issues, include activities that educate both sexes about the topics, first separately and then together in groups. For example, a cancer prevention program targeting women might also teach husbands about their wives' need for breast self-examination and Pap smears. Ideally, as they come to understand why and how these techniques are performed, some men may offer positive support and encouragement for their wives to practice these methods—or at least they may no longer interfere with their wives' practice of these methods.

6. *Identify positive role models from the community and train them to deliver your message or teach your program.* This method is used frequently in a variety of self-help programs in the health and mental health fields.

7. *Develop health education materials that use clear and simple language to reach people of all educational levels.* More information about materials development is presented in Chapter 4.

8. *Ask the members of the community to choose a name for the program so that it has special meaning to them.*

After you have done these things, be sure either to field-test your materials or to run a pilot of your program. Listen for people's comments or watch for their reactions. You may also want to conduct some focus groups to determine whether your ideas and strategies are appropriate and acceptable. They may also provide you with specific suggestions on how to revise your program or materials. Don't be discouraged if you need to make revisions. In fact, be prepared to make at least one revision, if not more, to your program or materials. This does not always mean your attempt was a failure; rather, it means that you are strengthening and improving your work!

¤ TRANSLATION: MORE THAN MEETS THE EYE

If you need to translate materials into other languages, consider carefully the method or methods you choose. Typically, there are three different techniques: one-way translation, translation by committee or consensus, and back-translation (sometimes referred to as *double translation*).

One-Way Translation

One-way translation depends on one bilingual individual to translate the original text into the second language. This is generally the method of choice for most people because it is both simple and economical. The problem with this method is that it assumes that one individual has the necessary comprehensive understanding of both languages and their cultural concepts to make a reliable translation. The mistakes or inaccuracies in the original text are not always identified, and this can lead to possible misinterpretations. Therefore, the result is often an awkward literal translation rather than one that represents the real meaning of the text. If you have no choice but to use this method, be sure to have the translation reviewed by other bilingual, bicultural individuals who reflect the diversity within your target group. For example, materials translated into Vietnamese should be reviewed by native speakers from the northern, central, and southern regions of Vietnam to make sure that they are easily understood by all. Also, field-test the one-way translation with individuals from the target group and discuss their understanding of the information. These suggestions will help strengthen the quality of a one-way translation.

Translation by Committee or Consensus

This method of translation uses two or more bilingual individuals to translate materials independently. Each translation is then reviewed, and differences are discussed among the translators to produce a consensus version. Because the translation does not rely solely on one individual's knowledge of both languages, the translation is more likely to be accurate. There are, however, some disadvantages to this method. First, it is more time-consuming and less economical. Also, if the translators do not reflect the diversity from within the community you are trying to reach, the translation may not be appropriate. For example, if you choose only professionals to translate, the translated material may be too difficult for your patients to understand or may not represent the vernacular of this group. In fact, this is a common problem even when you are writing in the same language. Finally, when trying to reach consensus, some of the translators may not feel comfortable contributing their ideas about the appropriateness of the translation. That is, one translator may defer to members of the committee who are older or more educated but not necessarily right. Therefore, your translation may appear to be a consensus version but actually conceal real disagreements about meaning. These limitations, however, can be avoided by (a) choosing a diverse group of translators from the target community and (b) allowing each to provide you with his or her written comments about the different translations before the consensus meeting. You or someone else can then facilitate the discussion about any noted disagreements. You may also want another person to review the consensus version, field-test it with some of your patients, or both.

Back-Translation

Back-translation requires at least two translators working independently. One translates the original material into the second language; the other takes this translated material and translates it back into the original language. The two original-language versions are then compared to identify significant differences. These differences are then discussed with the translators to determine the better alternative, or another round of back-translations can be done. This method has several advantages despite being more costly and time consuming. First, it allows for more than one interpretation of both the language and cultural concepts, thereby producing a more appropriate translation. This is especially so if more than one round of translations is done. Translators can meet to discuss differences in translation and any problems with regard to cultural relevance. Second, this method encourages each translator to treat his or her version as the original and discourages him or her from trying to infer meaning or make sense of a poor translation. At the time that each translator receives the material, ask each to identify words that could be translated in different ways or have different meanings, as well as any words or phrases that are awkward or nonsensical when translated. This allows you to consider alternative wording if regional differences exist in the second language. Again, the final translation should be field-tested. After the translation has been used and refined, consider modifying the original material so that it is linguistically more equivalent to the

TABLE 6.2 Tips on Writing Translatable English

Use simple language from the outset (grade-school level).

Use nouns rather than pronouns.

Avoid the use of metaphors or colloquial expressions (it is difficult to translate these and maintain the proper connotation).

Avoid possessive forms of words that may be misinterpreted when more than one actor is involved.

Use specific rather than general terms.

Avoid words that indicate vagueness about an event.

Use short and simple sentences (i.e., fewer than 16 words).

Use the active rather than the passive voice.

Avoid the subjunctive (e.g., verb forms with *would* or *could*).

Avoid adverbs and prepositions telling when and where (unless specific).

Avoid sentences with two different verbs if the verbs suggest different actions.

Use redundant wording to clarify the context and meaning of a phrase.

---

translated version. By doing this, you may improve the original text by making it less ambiguous in meaning or more easily understood. (Table 6.2 lists some tips on writing translatable English.)

The back-translation method is really the most reliable because it allows you to see the differences between the original and back-translated versions of the material. These differences, in turn, show you not only how the material has been translated but how it has been adapted so that it is culturally relevant.

◘ CONCLUSION

The creation of culturally relevant patient education programs is not an easy task but can be interesting and rewarding. We hope that the suggestions we have discussed in this chapter will help you approach this task more confidently, knowing that it involves careful research, planning, and, if possible, the collaboration of different people, especially the individuals you want to serve. It is their input that ensures the program's relevance and success. Although the suggestions presented here cannot guarantee your program's success, they certainly improve your chances for success and can help you establish a better working relationship with the different cultural groups in the future.

¤ BIBLIOGRAPHY

American Hospital Association. (1982). *Culture-bound and sensory barriers to communication with patients: Strategies and resources for health education.* Springfield, VA: National Technical Information Service.

Galanti, G.-A. (1997). *Caring for patients from different cultures: Case studies from American hospitals* (2nd cd.). Philadelphia, PA: University of Pennsylvania Press.

González, V. M., González, J. T., Freeman, V., & Howard-Pitney, B. (1991). *Health promotion in diverse cultural communities.* Stanford, CA: Stanford University Press.

Lynch, E. W., & Hanson, M. J. (Eds.). (1998). *Developing cross-cultural competence: A guide for working with children and their families.* Baltimore, MD: Brookes.

Purnell, L. D., & Paulenke, B. J. (Eds.). (1997). *Transcultural health care: A culturally competent approach.* Philadelphia, PA: F. A. Davis.

Randall-David, E. (1989). *Strategies for working with culturally diverse communities and clients.* Washington, DC: Association for the Care of Children's Health.

Selecting, Preparing, and Using Materials

Cecilia Doak
Leonard Doak
Lynn Gordon
Kate Lorig

Patient education materials can stand alone or can be used to supplement other types of patient education. They can be as simple as directions on how to take a medication or as complex as surgical procedures. They have value only if the materials accomplish what they are produced to accomplish. Therefore, a good place to start is to define the objectives and goals of your instruction.

Like all other aspects of patient education, materials should be produced on the basis of a needs assessment that results in specific objectives to be met by the materials (see Chapter 1). If you are working cross-culturally, you will need to learn about your target population and incorporate what you learn into any materials you produce (see Chapter 6). The value of educational materials is not judged by entertainment value or patient satisfaction. Rather, it is based on how well the materials meet their objectives (see Chapter 4).

When deciding to use materials, first decide whether you will use existing materials or create your own. Among the criteria for judging patient education material, three are especially important: (a) The material contains the information that the patient wants, (b) the material contains the information that the patient needs, and (c) the patient understands and uses the material as presented. Let us examine the application of these criteria.

¤ DOES THE MATERIAL CONTAIN THE INFORMATION THE PATIENT WANTS?

The only way to answer this question is by conducting a needs assessment before preparing or choosing material (see Chapter 1). Needs assessments may give you new insights into the appropriate use of material. For example, an assessment of people with asthma suggested that two problems often overlooked are anger and the stigma of having to use an inhaler in public. On the other hand, the needs assessment revealed that patients had little desire for more than very basic knowledge about how lungs function. Most asthma education materials do not address the problems of anger or the embarrassment caused by using an inhaler. They do, however, contain a great deal of information on pulmonary anatomy and physiology.

Another example was a needs assessment conducted with arthritis patients whose primary language was Spanish. They complained that it was very difficult for them to get good information about their disease. Materials written in English were not usable

TABLE 7.1 Health Care Professional Focus Versus Patient Focus

Health Care Professional Focus	*Patient Focus*
Anatomy and physiology (symptoms)	Why do I feel bad?
Necessary behaviors to maintain or improve health	Behaviors to solve problems caused by the disease
Facts about the disease	Beliefs about the disease
Skills necessary to carry out health-related behaviors	Skills necessary to maintain a "normal" life
Frustration that patients do not do what they should	Frustration/fear/depression about living with the disease
Fear about malpractice	Fear about the future

because of language. Health care providers did not speak Spanish or had very limited time. Finally, materials that were available in Spanish were simplified and brief. The Spanish-speaking patients wanted written materials that were clearly written, yet comprehensive. As a result of this assessment, the patient educators changed their plans from preparing a booklet in Spanish to writing a full-length book. Table 7.1 points out some of the different ways patients and health care professionals view the information contained in health materials. The material you prepare or choose should reflect the way patients think about health problems.

Needs assessments also provide us with information on how to frame our material. For example, we might use a question-and-answer format based on frequently asked patient questions or a problem-centered format based on patient problems. The importance of framing materials in the context of patient thinking rather than professional thinking cannot be overemphasized. A person recovering from a stroke will be more interested in "doing what you like" than in "your daily exercises."

Medical training teaches health care professionals to organize their knowledge according to the disease history, etiology, symptoms, treatment options, side effects, and so on. We refer to this content and sequence as the *medical model.* It may be suitable for health care professionals, but it is likely to be less effective for patient education. It does not focus on what most patients want and need to know.

Patients want to know what is wrong with them, what treatment can cure them, and when they can return to their normal lives. Other information such as success rate, treatment duration, and costs are also of interest. When you write instructions on behavior change, consider using the health belief model to organize the content and information sequence (see Chapter 2). Instructions written based on the HBM offer patients both the information they need and incentive to take the desired action. The differences between the medical model and a human behavior approach (the health belief model) are illustrated by the two versions of information on mammography shown in Table 7.2.

¤ DOES THE MATERIAL CONTAIN THE INFORMATION THE PATIENT NEEDS?

This question is not easy to answer. Most professionals think that they know what patients need to know. In fact, we are so sure we know what is best that we seldom question our assumptions. This can lead to some serious problems. For example, a young man facing a hip replacement was taught how to use a walker and how to use a backpack to move his belongings. Neither of these skills, however, prepared him to move his soup from the stove to the table.

To decide what information the patient needs to know, use the first two steps shown in the section headed "Setting Priorities" in Chapter 4. We need to ensure that the information is not too inclusive or exclusive. Sometimes, we put in too much and

TABLE 7.2 Comparison of Readability of Two Sets of Information on Mammography

Medical Model (readability: grade 12)	*Health Belief Model* (readability: grade 5)
An Extra Step: Mammography Women in the three high risk categories—age 50 or more, age 40 or more with a family history of breast cancer, age 35 or more with a personal history of breast cancer—may consider an additional routine screening method. This is x-ray mammography. Mammography uses radiation (x-rays) to create an image of the breast on film or paper called a mammogram. It can reveal tumors too small to be felt by palpation. It shows other changes in the structure of the breast which doctors believe point to very early cancer. A mammographic examination usually consists of two x-rays of each breast, one taken from the top and one from the side. Exposure to x-rays should always be carried out to assure that the lowest possible dose will be absorbed by the body. Radiologists are not yet certain if there is any risk from one mammogram, although most studies indicate that the risk, if it does exist, is small relative to the benefit. Recent equipment modifications and improved techniques are reducing radiation absorption and thus the possible risk.	**What is a mammogram and why should I have one?** A mammogram is an x-ray picture of the breast. It can find breast cancer that is too small for you, your doctor, or nurse to feel. Studies show that if you are in your forties or older, having a mammogram every 1 to 2 years could save your life. **How do I know if I need a mammogram?** Talk with your doctor about your chances of getting breast cancer. Your doctor can help you decide when you should start having mammograms and how often you should have them. **Why do I need a mammogram every 1 to 2 years?** As you get older, your chances of getting breast cancer get higher. Cancer can show up at any time—so one mammogram is not enough. Decide on a plan with your doctor and follow it for the rest of your life. **Where can I get a mammogram?** To find out where you can get a mammogram: • Ask your doctor or nurse • Ask your local health department or clinic • Call the National Cancer Institute's Cancer Information Service at 1-800-4-CANCER (1-800-422-6237).

SOURCE: National Cancer Institute, Bethesda, Maryland.

confuse the patient. In other cases, we do not supply all the information necessary to carry out the behaviors. For example, we usually tell patients when to take their medications, but we often forget to tell them what to do if they forget a dose or get off schedule. Instructions should include not only ideal circumstances but real circumstances as well.

¤ CAN THE PATIENT UNDERSTAND THE MATERIAL AS PRESENTED?

The best way to answer this question is to ask patients. Use questions that reveal comprehension, such as "What does this material tell you about _____ [subject]? What does it tell you to do?" Do not ask, "Do you understand?" because a yes answer does not tell you *what* they understand. Patients often say yes as an easy way to avoid more questions.

Too often, health professionals preempt patients and make decisions about what *they* think patients can or cannot understand. The most reliable way to find out whether material is understandable is to have representative patients or groups of patients use the material and give feedback on *what* they understand. This can be done through structured interviews or focus groups (see Chapter 1).

When we were writing a book for Spanish-speaking arthritis patients, we were concerned that there would be too much material or that the material would be at a level that was not easily understandable. But when we tested the book with a group of patients, we found a very different problem. The patients wanted more than one picture of each exercise. One drawing was not always enough for them to understand what to do. No one was concerned with the 200 pages of written text, even though some people in the test group had only a year or two of schooling.

These people told us that they wanted the information and that if they had a difficult time reading it, they would get help.

In short, there is no way around field testing. This is important whether you prepare your own material or choose materials that have been prepared by others. There is no shortage of patient education materials today. They are prepared by voluntary health associations such as the Cancer Society and the Lung Association. There are even materials for rarer conditions such as scleroderma and Gaucher disease. In addition, many commercial companies as well as drug companies publish patient education materials. The problem is choosing which ones are suitable for your patients. By applying the three criteria discussed, you will make this task easier.

One way to predict the ease or difficulty your patients may have with written material is to determine its literacy demand or its readability level. Is it likely to be too easy or over the heads of your intended audience? Readability formulas and the Suitability Assessment of Materials (SAM; Doak, Doak, & Root, 1995) are two means of determining this.

Readability Formulas

You can determine the readability of your material by using a simple formula based on just two factors: the number of words in the sentences and the number of syllables in the words. These factors predict the level of literacy needed for reading the material. Other tests such as the Cloze (Spadero, Robinson, & Smith, 1980) can indicate how well adults will understand specific patient education materials.

Why is it a good idea to test your material? Many health professionals write for patients as if they were writing for scientific journals. The application of a readability formula will help convince them that the material may not be understandable and needs to be revised. Most of all, a formula gives you an objective measure of the readability of your material. You can then judge how this might affect your audience. For example, if you are aiming material at people with an average of 4 years of formal education, university-level material will turn them off very quickly. Don't worry that good readers will feel talked down to by instructions with a low reading level. Research and experience show that adults at all reading skill levels prefer, remember better, and learn faster with easy-to-read instructions. An attainable goal for most health care instructions is the sixth-grade level. About 75% of adult Americans will be able to follow instructions reasonably well at this level.

Nearly all of the 40-plus different readability formulas provide a reasonably accurate grade level (typically plus or minus one grade level with a 68% confidence factor). We recommend the Fry formula, which covers levels from grade 1 through grade 17 (university level) and does not require an extensive test sample of the material (see Fry, 1968, 1977). More than a dozen computer programs are also available.

You do not have to test the readability of every word and sentence. Because reading levels may vary considerably from one part of your material to another, select three samples from different content topics, if possible. Select text only, not tables, figures, word lists, or graphics. (Figure 7.1 presents a graph for estimating readability, along with directions for use.)

Can the formulas in English be used for foreign languages? No—sentence construction, numbers of words with many syllables, and so forth vary markedly in different languages. Zakaluk and Samuels (1988) have published formulas in 11 different languages, but some have not been validated with large samples. The original purpose of readability formulas was for use in the elementary classroom to guide placement of students in developing reading skills.

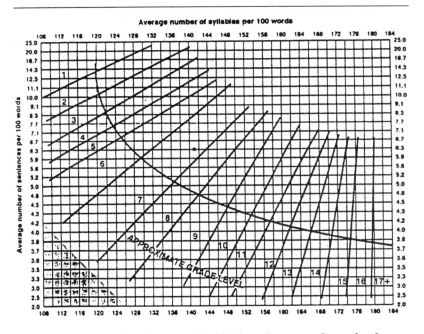

Directions: Randomly select 3 one hundred word passages from a book or an article. Plot average number of syllables and average number of sentences per 100 words on graph to determine the grade level of the material. Choose more passages per book of great variability is observed and conclude that the book has uneven readability. Few books will fall in a gray area but when they do grade levels are invalid.

Count proper nouns, numerals, and initialization as words. Count a syllable for each symbol. For example, 1945 is 1 word and 4 syllables and IRA is 1 word and 3 syllables.

Example:	*Syllables*	*Sentences*
1st hundred words	124	6.6
2nd hundred words	141	5.5
3rd hundred words	<u>158</u>	<u>6.8</u>
Average	141	6.3

Readability: 7th Grade (see dot plotted on graph)

Figure 7.1. Fry Graph for Estimating Readability–Extended

SOURCE: Fry (1977). Copyright © 1977 by the International Reading Association. Reprinted by permission.

The Suitability Assessment of Materials

To achieve understanding of our instructions, we have to work with much more than the readability of words and sentences. Let us examine the critical factors affecting the understanding process:

- The information presented should be what the patient wants and needs to know.
- The information needs to be at a readability level that the patient can read, and it is helpful if the material includes cues such as underlining, arrows, and highlighting to help guide the reader.
- Graphics and illustrations can provide learning enhancement and are powerful aids for remembering information.
- The layout of the page can make a great difference in whether the patient will read the material or ignore it.
- With very few exceptions, health care instructions are intended to be learned and to lead to specific behaviors. Instructions should be crafted so that they foster motivation and learning according to established learning theory.
- The material needs to be culturally suitable if it is to be accepted and adopted.

To help you apply these factors to your material, we present below a condensed version from the Suitability Assessment of Materials (Doak et al., 1995). Whether you are developing or evaluating health care materials, consider each of these factors:

1. Content
   a. Can patients easily understand the intended *purpose* of the material? If they cannot, they may not pay attention, or they may miss the main point.
   b. Is there clear, behavior-specific *content* that helps patients solve their problems? (For more discussion, see earlier sections of this chapter.)

c. Is the *scope* limited to the objectives? One problem with many materials is that they contain more information than patients need, want, or can reasonably learn.

d. Is there a *review* or *summary* of the key points? This is important, as readers often miss the key points on first exposure.

2. Literacy demands

a. Is the material written at an *appropriate readability level?* (See the discussion of readability formulas earlier in this chapter.)

b. Is the material presented in a *conversational style using the active voice?* Long or multiple phrases included in a sentence slow down the reading process and generally make comprehension more difficult.

c. Does the material use *common and explicit words?* For example:

- *doctor* rather than *physician*
- *use* rather than *utilize*
- *heart disease* rather than *coronary artery disease*
- *beans* rather than *legumes*
- *15-70* rather than *normal range*
- *pain lasting more than 5 minutes* rather than *excessive pain*

Whenever possible, use image words or analogies. These are things people can "see" or "feel." For example, *vegetables* is better than *dietary fiber,* and *a runny nose* is better than *excessive mucus.*

d. Is the *context* given before new information? We learn new facts/behaviors more quickly when told the context first: for example, "To find out what is wrong with you [the context first], the technician will take a sample of your blood for lab tests [new information]." (See Gopen & Swan, 1990.)

e. Are there *advance organizers* (road signs)? Headers or topic captions tell briefly what is coming up next. These advance organizers make material look less formidable and also prepare one's thought process to expect the next topic. They also help busy readers pick and choose what they want to read.

3. Graphics (illustrations, lists, tables, charts, graphs)

   a. Is the *cover graphic engaging?* Does it *convey* the message you want to convey? People do judge a booklet by its cover. This is a place to be especially careful. Does the cover graphic show what the material is all about?

   b. Are the *illustrations simple, realistic, and without distracting details?* Visuals are accepted and remembered better when they portray the familiar. Viewers may not recognize the meaning of medieval textbook drawings or abstract art or symbols. Photos should be limited in the amount of detail shown. Nonessential details such as room background, elaborate borders, and unnecessary color can be distracting.

   c. Do the illustrations tell the *key points* visually?

   d. Are all *graphics* (lists, tables, graphs, charts, geometric forms) *carefully and fully explained* in text near the graphic? Explanation and directions are essential and do little good if they are not in close proximity to the graphic.

   e. *Are captions used* to announce/explain graphics and illustrations? Captions can quickly tell the reader what the graphic or illustration is all about. A graphic without a caption is usually an inferior instruction and represents a missed learning opportunity. Keep in mind that captions should repeat or reinforce points from the text, not introduce new information.

4. Layout and typography

   a. *Are illustrations near related text?*

   b. Are there *visual cuing devices* such as boxes or arrows to point to the key information?

   c. Is there *adequate white space?* A cluttered page is hard to read.

   d. Does the material *look cluttered?*

   e. Is there *high color contrast* between the ink and the paper? (This is especially important for older people and those with visual problems.)

   f. Is the *print large enough?* If your readers will be over 40 or may not have fully corrected vision, use large type. If your readers will be people who need cataract surgery, use *much* larger type.

   g. Are more than six type fonts or sizes used on one page? Too many fonts and sizes make the material appear confusing.

   h. Are all CAPS used? Type in all capital letters slows down reading comprehension for readers at all skill levels (see White, 1988).

   i. Are there more than five to seven items on a list? Few people can remember more than seven independent items. For adults with lower literacy skills, the limit may be three to five items. Longer lists need to be partitioned into smaller chunks (see Miller, 1956).

5. Learning stimulation motivation

   a. *Is interaction included in the text or graphic?* Readers/viewers should be asked to *do something* (solve problems, make choices, demonstrate, and so on).

   b. Are desired *behaviors shown in specific terms* and modeled? People learn more readily by observation and doing rather than by reading or being told.

   c. *Are the behaviors presented as doable?* People are more motivated when they believe the tasks are doable. Telling people with emphysema to "exercise" is not very motivating. Telling them that "everyone can walk 10 minutes a day by walking 1 minute for each hour that he or she is awake" is much more motivating.

6. Cultural appropriateness

   a. Do the language, logic, experience, and illustrations *match* the language, logic, and experience of the population? For example, are the foods, activities, and home remedies mentioned familiar to your intended readers? Do the pictures look like the people who will be using the material?

   b. *Are the cultural images positive, realistic, and appropriate?* Using Grandma Moses as an example of successful aging may be meaningless to a Hispanic population.

   c. *Does the material convey respect?* There is a tendency to infantilize materials for people from other cultures. People with

low literacy and those who speak a language other than the
society's dominant one have the same ability to learn as
others, if they are taught appropriately. Convey respect not
only with words but also with high-quality production. You
don't need to use glossy paper and pop-ups; the main thing
is that your materials be written, illustrated, and produced
with care.

The above list was developed to evaluate materials that are
already written. It can also be used as a guide when preparing
new materials. A word of caution, however: This is not a tem-
plate for preparing materials. Rather, it is a guide. Read it over,
prepare your materials, and then check them out to see if you
have missed anything important.

◘ SUMMARY

A key point covered in this chapter is that patients and health
professionals see instructional needs differently. In preparing
materials, we often focus on what we want the patient to know.
This chapter broadens our perspective to include what the patient wants to know as well as how to organize our information so
that our advice is easier to understand and carry out. Several suggestions are offered to help balance what we know is important
with what the patient seems to want. In summary:

- Try to involve the patient in all stages of design of educational
  materials.
- Apply sound health education theory in selection of content and
  in the organization and prioritization of the information (e.g.,
  consider the health belief model).
- Ask yourself the detailed questions listed under each of six SAM
  topics above. The questions go far beyond factors such as readability and into the dynamics of the comprehension and learning

processes (e.g., visuals and graphics, motivation, and cultural factors).

The consequences of selecting an unsuitable approach are serious: The patient may not understand the material or may ignore it. This chapter offers a blueprint for the development of effective materials that will be suitable for your patients.

✪ BIBLIOGRAPHY

Doak, C., Doak, L., & Root, J. H. (1995). *Teaching patients with low literacy skills* (2nd ed.). Philadelphia, PA: J. B. Lippincott.

Fry, E. (1968). A readability formula that saves time. *Journal of Reading, 2,* 513-516, 575-578.

Fry, E. (1977). Fry's Readability Graph: Clarification, validity, and extension to level 17. *Journal of Reading, 11,* 242-252.

Gopen, G. D., & Swan, J. A. (1990). The science of scientific writing. *American Scientist, 78,* 550-558.

Miller, G. A. (1956). The magical number seven, plus or minus two: Some limits on our capacity for processing information. *Psychological Review, 63,* 81-87.

Spadero, D. C., Robinson, L. A., & Smith, L. A. (1980). Assessing readability of patient education materials. *American Journal of Hospital Pharmacy, 37,* 215-221.

White, J. V. (1988). *Graphic design for the electronic age: The manual for traditional and desktop publishing.* New York: Watson-Guptil.

Zakaluk, B. L., & Samuels, S. J. (1988). *Readability: Its past, present, and future.* Newark, DE: International Reading Association.

8

Helping People Who Are Hard to Help

Kate Lorig

One of the greatest challenges in patient education is dealing with people who are hard to help. Fortunately, there are a limited number of problems that seem to appear over and over again. Once you recognize them and their solutions, dealing with them becomes much easier. In this chapter, you will meet some of the most common types of problem people and learn ways of helping them.

¤ STRONG, SILENT TYPES

One of the greatest fears of patient educators is that they will not be able to get people to ask questions or to discuss topics. There is also a strongly held belief that "people here are different. They don't talk." "Here" can mean any region, country, or culture.

People are not really all that different. Rather, it is some patient educators who are insecure about their own knowledge and abilities, and who never really invite participation. Usually, they give a talk and then ask if there are any questions. Given 10 seconds and no response, they decide that there are no questions and continue or end the session.

If you are trying to get participation, several techniques will be very helpful. You might present a problem or question, such as "What would you do if . . . ?" Have all the participants write down their answers and then go around the room, having each participant tell what he or she wrote. This technique ensures that everyone participates in a nonthreatening way. But in using this technique, first be sure that the question is one that is nonthreatening and with which the participants have experience—for example, "What is the greatest problem in controlling your diet?" When using this technique, the leader should start by modeling an appropriate response using a personal experience. Please note that your modeling is very important. If you tell a long story, expect everyone else in the class to do the same thing. If, on the other hand, you are brief and to the point, participants will follow your lead. Finally, start with a participant who you know will be able to respond. Once the group is clear on the expectation and knows that responses will be handled in a nonjudgmental way, generally everyone will follow.

A second way of getting group participation is to brainstorm. Some details on using this technique are discussed in Chapter 4.

When asking the group questions, be sure that your questions ares open-ended. A good rule to follow is never to ask a question that can be answered by yes or no. "What questions do you have?" is better than "Are there any questions?" Then, after asking for questions, count to 30 slowly. Groups do not like silence, and someone will generally say something to fill the void.

If the silence makes you uncomfortable, you can add a second prompt such as "Surely there are some questions?" Once the ice is broken, more questions and discussion usually follow.

Make the group safe for questions and discussions. Give reinforcement to everyone who participates with smiles, nods of your head, or positive comments such as "That is a good question" or "I'm so glad you asked that. Many people have the same problem and are afraid to discuss it." Be careful not to make participants feel stupid or silly. Even if you get a bizarre comment, respond with a noncommittal, neutral statement such as "That's an interesting comment" or "I see your point of view."

By using the techniques described above, you can almost always get good group participation. However, there may still be some nonparticipating group members. First, be sure that these people are sitting in the group. Often, they will place themselves physically outside the group. If someone is a chronic nonparticipant, address questions directly to him or her—for example, "Jim/Maria, what do you think about that?" Be sure that you do not put the nonparticipant on the spot, however. Always ask something that you know he or she can answer.

Sometimes, you will have situations in which husbands or wives answer for their spouses or parents answer for their child. In these cases, address your questions directly to the child or silent spouse. If someone else answers, say, "No, let Jill speak for herself." Then be patient and let this happen. Be especially sure to reinforce any participation by your strong, silent types. In addition, watch them carefully for any sign that they might like to participate but are holding back. A change in posture or facial expression or a slightly raised finger may be all the clue you get. Do not miss this.

In almost every class, you will have a sleeper. Do not let this worry you. Just let the person sleep—he or she is probably tired. It has nothing to do with your presentation. If more than 25% of the class is sleeping, then you might be the problem. However, if the class is made up of medical students or doctors, even a 50% sleep rate is acceptable.

A final point about nonparticipation: You must really want participation and schedule time for it. I recently observed a patient educator who complained that people in his class would not ask questions. What really happened was this: He asked for questions, and two hands went up. He called on one person and then spent 10 minutes in a one-to-one dialogue with this person on a topic that was not of general interest to the class. He then proceeded with his lecture, never getting back to the other person who had a question. It is not difficult to see why people hesitated to participate.

¤ TALKERS

Once you have gotten your group to participate, the problem will probably be shutting them up. Too much participation can be just as bad as no participation; this takes skill to control. Here are some situations that might arise.

Participants come to a course with some special problems or questions. They often want these answered right away. As a leader, you can easily be thrown from your agenda by trying to meet participants' needs immediately. Do not be afraid to say, "We are going to discuss medications in the third session; right now we are discussing exercise" or "That is a little off the topic, but I will be pleased to discuss it with you over coffee. Right now, it is important to get on with the class." To help keep such situations from occurring, you should have an agenda posted at the start of each class, divided into topics and showing the time allotted to each. Then, if you are behind, you can point to the agenda as a reason for charging ahead.

One of the most troublesome of all class participants is the talker. He or she almost always has something to say, which usually includes a long story. Sometimes talkers' stories and insights are useful and relevant; other times, they are useless. In either case, the person who usurps time must be controlled. One way to do this is simply to avoid calling on the person. But this is of limited usefulness, because often this person will just butt in, asked or not. Sometimes you have to be very blunt: "Your opinions are helpful, but others need a chance to be heard." This may seem harsh and unfeeling; however, such a statement is usually handled with good grace. The people who hog time know when they are being "hoggish." Sometimes, you can use the seating arrangement to control this situation. If you sit next to the talker, it is more difficult for him or her to get your attention and cut in.

Another frequent problem is when a participant rambles on and on, even though the point of the story, if there is a point, was made in the first 15 seconds. In this case, the only thing to do is cut the person off. Wait until he or she takes a breath—it has to happen sometime—and quickly say, "Thank you very much." Immediately call on someone else or start a new activity. At the same time, physically turn away from the person.

Side talkers are very common. These are people who are always chatting to their neighbors. To begin with, ask them to be quiet. If this does not work, try sitting between the two friends. This is sometimes successful. If not, a little sarcasm might be helpful: "If you two don't stop talking, I'll have to ask one of you to stand in the corner."

There is one special case of talker. People who arrive late almost always try to "make up" for their lateness with immediate participation. This participation may be inappropriate or even destructive. You can sidetrack this a bit by helping to integrate the person. For example, "Joe, we were worried about you. I'm glad you're here. We were just discussing . . . ."

On very rare occasions, you will find a whole class that is very difficult to control. They all talk at once. In this case, seating can come to your rescue. Although we generally like to have small groups sit in a circle, arranging people in rows, at desks or with tables in front of them, tends to reestablish control and quiet discussion. If all else fails, rearrange the room. Of course, if the problem is lack of participation in a formal setting, try making the setting less formal.

✪ ANTAGONISTIC OR BELLIGERENT PARTICIPANTS

Fortunately, antagonistic or belligerent people do not appear too often. They, too, can be helped. The first thing to remember is not to argue with them—this just leads to more argument. Instead, try something like this: "I understand your beliefs, but our current knowledge in this suggests . . ." or "If you find that eating fish cures your ulcers, then please continue eating fish. However, for most people, we find that _____ will be more helpful."

Sometimes, a leader and a participant will argue with each other. Somehow, whatever the leader says adds more antagonism. When this happens, it is usually a play for power by someone who is used to being the center of attention. One way to help this situation is to place the powermonger out of direct eye contact with the leader. In a circle, the best way of doing this is to place the person next to the leader. Somehow, being out of eye contact tends to defuse the situation.

If all else fails, you may have to ask the belligerent person to leave the class. You can do this by saying, "I don't think this class will meet your needs. If you will see me during coffee or call me tomorrow, we can see if we can find something more suitable." At this point, the belligerent person may leave. More likely, he or she will simmer down and participate more appropriately. In either case, things will be easier for you and for participants.

✪ "YES, BUTS"

Some people always have an excuse for not doing what you ask. They are usually easy to identify by their distinctive call, "Yes, but . . ." After hearing two or three "yes, buts," give up. An easy rule of thumb is this: Three "yes, buts" and they are out. There is no way you can help them by acting helpfully. Instead, confront them:

> I know that you have many problems. However, the decision
> to do something or not is yours. I do not have high blood pres-
> sure, so it is not my problem. If you want to do something, fine;
> I will try to be helpful. If not, that is okay too. It is your choice.

Such a statement makes it very clear where the problem lies and
that it is up to the individual to take responsibility. Do not spend
all your time with these people. You probably will not be able to
help them. In trying to help them, you deny help to others who
are more ready to act. One of the best ways of turning a "Yes,
But" around is to ignore him or her. Often, when someone gets
attention for action rather than nonaction, you see a change in
his or her behavior.

The "Know-It-All" is just a variation of the "Yes, But." This
person knows all the answers and has tried everything. There is
nothing you can teach him or her. Acknowledge that the person
is very knowledgeable and that you might not be able to teach
him or her anything. Then give the individual the choice of continuing with the group or leaving. Most of the time, once his or
her game is called, the person will become an active and helpful
participant. Sometimes he or she will leave, and this is okay too.

¤ ATTENTION SEEKERS

We have already talked about several types of attention seekers—the Belligerents, the Know-It-Alls, and the "Yes, Buts."
There are two more types that, unfortunately, have a high preva-
lence in patient education classes.

The "Whiners" are those people with a million problems.
Sometimes, they are also "Yes, Buts." Somehow, they manage to
get the whole class involved in the catastrophe they call life.
Everyone feels sorry for them. Often their stories are truly traumatic—they were molested as children, have alcoholic husbands,
or are about to get evicted from the family home. Besides, no one
loves them. First, you must remember that their stories may or

may not be true. Second, there are probably three or four other people in the class with equally wrenching lives who somehow are coping and productive. If you and the class get bogged down with Whiners, no one wins and everyone loses. Instead, suggest that you will talk with them during the coffee break or after class and try to make some appropriate referrals. Do not spend class time trying to solve their problems!

The second group of attention seekers plays a game called "My disease is worse than your disease." They seek status by laying claim to the worst disease. It is important to cut this game short at the beginning. Statements such as the following may help:

> In this class, everyone has problems with _____. Some of these may seem worse than others, but you can never judge another by your standard. The paraplegic in a loving family may get along very well, whereas the loss of a finger can be devastating to a concert violinist. In this class, we will try to help everyone with his or her problems and not make judgments about the severity of the problems.

Another way of cutting short this disease status game is not to let participants give their disease history or to describe themselves in terms of the disease. This is especially important in introductions. See how this is handled in the Chronic Disease Self-Management Workshop in Appendix 4B, in Chapter 4. Ask people to tell about their families or hobbies, about what they want to get out of the course, or about the problems caused by their condition. *Do not* ask them to tell about their disease.

✿ SPECIAL PROBLEM PEOPLE

Two final types of problem people are not very common but need to be recognized and dealt with quickly: the "ists" and the "inappropriates."

The "ists" are the people who are racists, sexists, or ageists. They are the men who call women "girls," the women who make negative statements about men, the young people who make rude remarks about older people, and the people who sprinkle their language with racist, sexist, and ageist slurs. Any time you encounter an "ist," you should make it clear that such language and thinking do not have a place in the class setting. This is true even if you do not have members of the "ist's" targeted race, ethnicity, gender, or age in your class.

In some ways, the "inappropriates" are the easiest to handle. These are the people who clearly have mental health problems that are usually obvious in the first few minutes of the class. If their speech and behavior are not disruptive, then let them stay. However, if they are in any way disruptive, then help them find a more appropriate setting to work on their problems. It is not fair to the rest of the class or to the "inappropriates" to keep such persons around.

This chapter has addressed the most common types of problem people. Sometimes, you may encounter other problems or groups of people with multiple problems. In such cases, seek some help. A psychologist or social worker who has experience with group work can be an excellent resource. When you are in trouble, do not be afraid to ask for help.

9

The Special Problem
of Compliance
How Do I Get People to
Do What Is Good for Them?

Kate Lorig

Various researchers have estimated that people comply with
new health behaviors 30%-70% of the time. Taken at face value,
this paints a sorry picture and suggests that compliance is a major
problem. However, it is necessary to examine this issue a bit
more closely.

For some health-related regimes, compliance is a very important issue. We know that it is necessary for many people to
take insulin daily in order to control diabetes. However, we do
not have any similar data to suggest the exact type, amount, or
duration of exercise necessary either to prevent or to overcome

the musculoskeletal problems caused by arthritis. Much of arthritis treatment is physical therapy practice, common sense,
and clinical experience. However, it is not backed by strong scientific evidence. When such evidence is lacking, it is difficult
to justify the importance of exact compliance with an exercise
program.

Another issue involves the interactions between the disease
and the desired health behaviors. For many diseases, the symptoms wax and wane on almost a daily basis. Therefore, the
lockstep continuation of a set of behaviors in the face of changing
symptoms does not seem to make a great deal of sense. Rather
than demonstrating strict compliance, a person must understand
the rationale for his or her program and also know how to make
daily adjustments in the face of these changing symptoms. If this
is not done, behavior change becomes a frustrating experience
in which the patient either exacerbates the symptoms or gets no
therapeutic effect because the intervention is not tailored to the
symptoms. Balancing behavior change with symptoms takes
knowledge, practice, and, most important, decision-making skills.
Unfortunately, health professionals seldom teach decision-making skills in traditional interactions with patients. (For further
reading on this topic, see Cramer & Spilder, 1991; Mager & Pipe,
1970; Sackett & Haynes, 1976.)

On the basis of the above discussion, it would seem that specific compliance may not always be a desired or even a necessary
behavior. A more appropriate goal might be adherence to a
long-term program with constant changes in response to symptoms. However, even with this broader definition, it is doubtful
that most people would adopt new programs appropriately. The
rest of this chapter addresses some reasons for inappropriate
compliance patterns and suggests some ways of identifying
problems with individual patients as well as some techniques for
solving these problems. The terms *compliance* and *adherence* are
used interchangeably here.

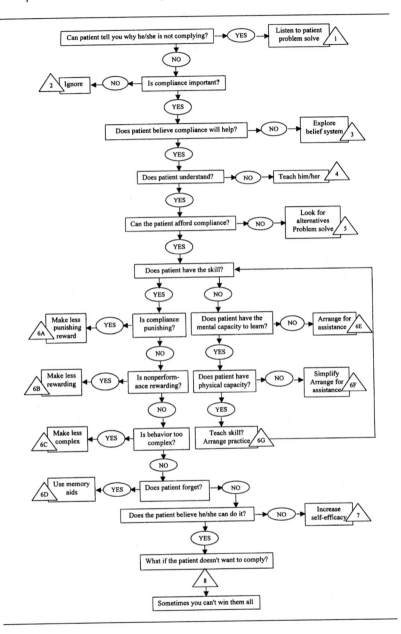

Figure 9.1. Improving Patient Compliance

Let us now turn to exploring how to help people with compliance. The decision flowchart displayed in Figure 9.1 shows a series of questions you can ask. Start at the top of the chart and work through it until you find a description of the problem you are encountering. Each level of the chart lists one or more actions that might be taken in the boxes next to the triangles. Look up further discussion of these actions in the text that follows by referring to the numbers given in the triangles.

1. Can the patient tell you why he or she is not complying?

This may seem like an obvious question. However, all too often we forget to ask. When we do ask, the patient will usually tell us the problem. The normal response of most professionals when confronted with a patient problem is to offer the patient a solution. This is probably not the best response. Rather, this is an ideal time to teach problem-solving skills. To do this, ask the patient to brainstorm possible solutions. For example, if a patient says she does not have enough time to exercise in the morning, ask when else in the day she might have 10 minutes to do her exercises. If a patient says he forgets to exercise, ask about activities that he does daily, such as reading the morning paper or watching a favorite TV show, and then link the exercises to one such activity. The moral here is that most patients can tell you the problem and, with a little assistance, come up with a solution. Never underestimate your patient.

2. Is compliance important?

This may seem like a silly question. However, as discussed earlier, we really do not know exactly which exercise program is best for which patient. The result is that we often ask patients to do things that may not be important. For example, are daily range-of-motion exercises necessary for every stroke patient? The answer is probably no. In fact, range-of-motion exercise three or four times a week is probably sufficient. Do all joints need to be put through a daily range-of-motion exercise? Again, the answer is probably no. One needs to exercise only those joints in which there is some limitation. If compliance is not important, then forget about it. Both you and the patient have more important things to worry about.

3. Does your patient believe that compliance will help? (No)

If the answer to this question is no, then the reason for non-compliance is obvious. Why should anyone do anything in which he or she does not believe? Although the problem may be obvious, the solution is a bit more difficult. People's beliefs are almost always rational and based on culture, past experience, conversations with others, what they have been taught, or any combination of those factors. Often, it is the use of language that leads patients to false beliefs. Arthritis health professionals often talk about osteoarthritis as a "wear-and-tear disease." It is not. When patients hear this characterization, they easily translate it into rational action: "Why should I exercise if my disease is caused by wear and tear? Exercise increases the problem." One of the ways to help to change beliefs is to change the use of language. Avoid using the incorrect wear-and-tear explanation for osteoarthritis.

Another means of changing beliefs is to expand on the patient's current belief system. If someone believes that pain is due to disease, then he or she is likely to believe also that the way to counter the pain must be through medical interventions such as medication. However, if you can expand the explanation of pain to include not only disease but muscle tension, fear, and depression, then the patient may try other pain management modalities, such as exercise and relaxation.

Finding out patients' beliefs is not difficult–ask them. Good questions include the following: "What do you think causes your pain?" "Why is exercise important?" "When you think of diabetes, what do you think of?" Before you give any explanation, it is important to find out what the patient already knows and believes. In this way, teaching is targeted and time is not wasted (for more about beliefs, see the section on salient beliefs assessment in Chapter 1).

4. Does the patient understand? (No)

Do not believe that patients understand just because they say they do. This is especially true with medication regimes. It is one thing to repeat what the doctor says and quite another to integrate medication taking into one's life. If people are not sure of what they are doing, they will often do nothing rather than risk doing something wrong. Another problem is that we often give instructions only for the ideal case–for example, "Take this medication twice a day." We do not tell patients what to do in real cases–for example, "If you miss one dose, take it as soon as you remember. Do not double up doses."

Whenever you give patients instructions, take four steps to ensure understanding. First, tell patients what you want them to do in plain language. Forget the use of terms such as *TID*. Second, if you want patients to exercise, show them what you want them to do and have them return the demonstration until they can do the procedure easily without coaching. Third, give patients written instructions, including, if necessary, pictures. Finally, ask patients to describe what they are going to do. Do not accept a parroting of your original explanation. Rather, ask questions such as "When are you going to take your medicine, and how many pills will you take each time?" In short, TWA– tell, write, ask.

5. Can the patient afford compliance?

This question has two parts. First, can the patient afford the cost? If the answer is no, then we must do something to help. Sometimes, medications can be changed to less expensive ones. Also, we can help patients find less expensive ways of buying drugs, such as from on-line services. There may be times that we have to help patients get some form of public assistance. Here, the educational issue is to inform patients of alternatives.

In some cases, the patient cannot afford the time for compliance. For example, a busy mother with four children may not believe it is possible to walk for an hour a day. In such a case, your problem solving with the patient may lead her to use her time in some alternative ways, such as walking the dog to the grocery store or getting a piece of exercise equipment that can be used at home.

6. Does the patient have the skill to comply? (Yes)

6A. Is compliance punishing? (Yes)

In many cases, complying with health regimes is not only nonrewarding but punishing. For example, many drugs have side effects, diets take away pleasures, and exercise may leave one stiff. Each of these cases is a bit different, but the solution is similar: Make compliance less punishing and more rewarding. When compliance means physiological punishment, such as stiffness from exercise, symptom reinterpretation is useful (see more about this in Chapter 2 in the section on self-efficacy). Explain that the stiffness means that the treatment is actually doing some good. The patient might interpret stiffness as meaning that the exercise is causing worsening of the disease.

In another case, exercise might be punishing because of the time of day or weather conditions. Few people like to walk a mile before breakfast on a cold winter day. In this case, another time might be found, or a warm place, such as a shopping mall, or even an alternate exercise, such as riding a stationary bicycle.

6B. Is nonperformance rewarding? (Yes)

Sometimes noncompliance brings rewards such as attention, albeit in a nagging form, from spouses or friends. Also, the short-term rewards of noncompliance, such as remaining in bed on a cold morning, might outweigh the long-term rewards of a daily early-morning walk. If noncompliance is rewarding, the best thing to do is to remove the reward. Ignoring noncompliance may be difficult but may also be the best way to bring about improvement. This is especially true with couples between whom sometimes the only communication is nagging. Reestablishing more positive communication patterns may be the answer.

6C. Is the behavior too complex? (Yes)

Sometimes we ask patients to do many things all at the same time. They are taking several medications, are on a special diet, and have three sets of exercises to perform daily. In addition, they are asked to have appointments with one or more health professionals on a regular basis. Is it any wonder that they don't comply? Before talking to patients about compliance, it is important to get the whole picture of what they are trying to do. Ask them, "What are all the things that various people have told you to do?" These may range from flossing their teeth to drinking warm milk before going to bed every night. What you want them to do is only a small part of the total picture and, compared with some other activities, may be relatively unimportant. In any case, as a health professional, you have the job of sorting out the jumble and simplifying the regime. This may mean contacting other health professionals to see which of their instructions are really important. In some cases, instructions may even be contradictory. For example, the rheumatologist says to limit weight-bearing exercise because of bad knees, but the cardiologist says to forget the knees and walk as much as possible. The patient loses no matter what he or she does. Once you and the patient understand the whole regime, priorities can be set and complexities simplified.

6D. Does the patient forget? (Yes)

Patient forgetfulness is probably one of the greatest causes of noncompliance. It is not easy to add new activities to our lives, especially if these activities must be performed more than once a day. Memory aids, such as setting an alarm clock or a wristwatch alarm, can remind patients when it is time for them to take medications. Medicine bottles can now be purchased with built-in alarms.

Another and more powerful memory aid is to link the new behavior with an already established activity. For example, range-of-motion exercises can be done in the morning shower, and a walk can be taken before lunch. Medication can be taken when brushing teeth. Most of us are creatures of habit. The easiest way to establish a new habit is to link it with an existing habit. Those who are cognitively impaired may need more help. A sample of all pills and the times they are to be taken can be posted on a board. Then the day's pills can be laid out below the sample. The patient need only look at the board to find out if he or she has taken the pill. Using this method, the patient might be able to lay out his or her own pills each day.

6E. Does the patient have the mental capacity to learn the skill? (No)

If the answer to this question is no, you might try some of the tricks we discussed as memory aids. However, it is more likely that you will need to find someone to assist the patient. This might be a spouse or other family member, a neighbor, or possibly a home health aide or visiting physical therapist. Many older people who live alone are part of an informal helping network of friends and neighbors. Such networks are especially helpful for the cognitively impaired. Is there someone who can call twice a day to remind the patient to do something? Maybe there is a neighbor who will take a daily walk with the patient or assist with medication taking. In any case, the answer is usually to find some assistance.

6F. Does the patient have the physical capacity to do the skill? (No)

If the answer to this question is no, then there are several routes to take. First, the activity might be simplified or changed to bring it within the physical capacity of the patient. See 6C, above, for suggestions on how to make activities less complex. On the other hand, the patient may need assistance. The suggestions under 6E might be helpful.

6G. Teach skill and arrange practice and feedback.

If the patient does not have the skill but has the cognitive and physical capacity to learn the skill, then the tricks to compliance are teaching, practice, and feedback. First, the patient must be taught the skill. This can sometimes be done verbally or in writing. However, if there is any unusual physical skill involved, then teaching must include demonstration and practice. For instance, one cannot learn to ride a bicycle from reading a book, and it is not realistic to expect patients to learn to inject insulin from written materials. Rather, patients need an opportunity for supervised practice and feedback. It is especially important that during the demonstration, patients do the whole activity without assistance. This may be very frustrating for the health professional. However, the important thing is that patients leave the teaching session confident that they can do the activity themselves. Remember that even the most complex behavior can be broken down into simple, achievable parts.

The final part of teaching a skill is arranging for feedback. This can be provided as part of the demonstration or return demonstration. Compliance is even more likely if patients have a way of getting their questions answered and receiving feedback when they are at home. This can often be provided by telephone. Another possibility is sending patients home with a video so that they can review the procedure.

7. Does the patient believe that he or she can do it? (No)

This is probably the key to many compliance problems. Just because people know how to do something and even have the required skills does not mean they believe they can do it. Many people who are overweight believe that this condition is harmful, know all about exercise and low-calorie food, and even know how to exercise and eat appropriately. However, all these beliefs and knowledge are not enough because these people do not believe themselves capable of carrying out the program and losing weight. Bandura (1982) calls this belief in one's ability to carry out specific behaviors *perceived self-efficacy*. In this case, your job is to increase the patient's confidence. See the section on self-efficacy in Chapter 2.

8. What if the patient does not want to comply?

Just because you want patients to do something and know that it is good for them, that is no reason they have to agree. Patients have a right to make their own decisions for their own reasons. You should be convinced that the decision is informed. That is, that patients understand your rationale for wanting them to do something. Once this criterion is met, if patients still decide not to comply, you should honor their decision. Health professionals have a limited amount of time. Often, time is wasted trying to work with patients who have no intention of changing. More important, it deprives other patients who can be helped of the health professional's time. Sometimes, the best thing to do is just let a patient go. If this occurs, make it very clear to the patient what you are doing. For example: "Mrs. Jones, I understand that you do not want to exercise. We have discussed the various reasons that exercise might be good for you. However, I do respect your decision. If in the future I can help you with an exercise program, please let me know." This statement does several things. First, it lets Mrs. Jones know that the decision not to exercise is hers. Second, it leaves the door open should she change her mind. Finally, it shows your respect for her, even though you disagree with her decision.

In short, if people do not want to comply, you cannot make them. Sometimes, you just can't win them all.

✸ BIBLIOGRAPHY

Bandura, A. (1982). Self-efficacy in human agency. *American Psychologist, 37,* 122-147.

Cramer, J. A., & Spilder, B. (Eds.). (1991). *Patient compliance in medical practice and clinical trials.* New York: Raven.

Mager, R. F., & Pipe, P. (1970). *Analyzing performance problems.* Belmont, CA: Fearon.

Sackett, D. L., & Haynes, R. B. (1976). *Compliance with therapeutic regimes.* Baltimore, MD: Johns Hopkins University Press.

10

Meeting JCAHO Standards for Patient Education

Barbara E. Giloth

The year 1994 marked the first time that the Joint Commission on Accreditation of Healthcare Organizations (JCAHO) included a separate chapter on patient and family education in its *Accreditation Manual for Hospitals.* The standards contained in that chapter were built based on key publications from the late 1970s, such as *A Model for Patient Education Programming* (Deeds, Hebert, & Wolle, 1979) and *Implementing Patient Education in the Hospital* (American Hospital Association, 1979), and, more recently, *Managing Hospital-Based Patient Education* (Giloth, 1993). Up until 1994, references to patient education were scattered throughout discipline-specific and setting-specific chapters in the JCAHO manual. Whether or not patient education was addressed during a survey depended on the interest of surveyor. Hospital patient education staff were rarely, if ever, asked to participate in the survey interviews. The 1994 changes have made a big difference to some hospital staff who did not know about, or chose to ignore, the importance of patient and family education. Of course, staff members responsible for patient education have always understood the importance of interdisciplinary coordination and management.

During the past decade, the JCAHO standards have undergone another major transformation. They are now performance-based, functionally organized standards. Less emphasis is now placed on *how* to achieve the intent of a given standard—the goal is to reach specified outcomes. This is achieved through the creative development of structures and processes that meet the unique needs of each organization and its patients. The new approach has also moved from evaluating specific departments and services to assessing the performance of interdisciplinary functions throughout the organization.

The major focus on patient education within the current accreditation manual falls in the "Education" chapter in the first section of the volume, which is titled "Patient-Focused Functions" (JCAHO, 1999). The standards are listed here in Table 10.1. They address the need for a systematic approach to education and also serve as the basis for the accreditation interviews of both staff and patients. Table 10.1 also includes cross-references to earlier chapters in this book that can be helpful to you in meeting the intent of specific standards. Although much of the content of this book is oriented toward developing education programs for groups of patients, the same planning principles are recognized by accreditation surveyors as necessary for the development of teaching resources. This planning process is also compatible with your individualizing target population programs to specific patients. The chapters here addressing work with cross-cultural populations, special concerns in working with challenging patients, and compliance issues (Chapters 6, 8, and 9, respectively) will also help you with the individualization process.

text continues on page 225

TABLE 10.1 JCAHO Education Standards and Corresponding Helpful Chapters in This Volume

JCAHO Education Standard	Helpful Chapters in This Book
PF.1. The patient's learning needs, abilities, preferences, and readiness to learn are assessed.	See especially Chapter 1, "How Do I Know What Patients Want and Need?" and Chapter 3, "Do I Know Where to Go, and Will I Know When I Get There?" for approaches to gathering information about needs. Chapter 2, "What Do We Know About What Works?" describes how different models can help to pinpoint important patient concerns and barriers to change. Chapter 7, "Selecting, Preparing, and Using Materials," helps staff evaluate whether or not teaching materials are understood by patients. Finally, Chapter 9, "The Special Problem of Compliance," offers a helpful algorithm to identify and solve compliance problems.
PF.1.1. The assessment considers cultural and religious practices, emotional barriers, desire and motivation to learn, physical and cognitive limitations, language barriers, and the financial implications of care choices.	See especially Chapter 6, "Working Cross-Culturally," and Chapter 8, "Helping People Who Are Hard to Help." Additionally, Chapter 2, "What Do We Know About What Works?" provides insight into motivation and barriers to learning, and Chapter 7, "Selecting, Preparing, and Using Materials," offers strategies to use with low-literacy learners.
PF.1.2. When called for by the age of the patient and the length of stay, the hospital assesses and provides for patients' academic education needs.	Although this standard is broadly addressed in Chapter, "How Do I Know What Patients Want and Need?" the topic is not really covered in depth in this book.

continued

221

TABLE 10.1 Continued

JCAHO Education Standard	Helpful Chapters
PF.1.3. Patients are educated about the safe and effective use of medication, according to law and their needs.	Although specific content information is not provided, many of the chapters here address the challenges of providing education to patients, including Chapter 2, "What Do We Know About What Works?"; Chapter 4, "How Do I Get From a Needs Assessment to a Program?"; Chapter 7, "Selecting, Preparing, and Using Materials"; Chapter 6, "Working Cross-Culturally"; and Chapter 9, "The Special Problem of Compliance." Chapter 3, "Do I Know Where to Go, and Will I Know When I Get There?" provides guidance on how to find out whether the teaching objectives have been met.
PF.1.4. Patients are educated about the safe and effective use of medical equipment.	
PF.1.5. Patients are educated about potential drug-food interactions and provided counseling on nutrition and modified diets.	
PF.1.6. Patients are educated about rehabilitation techniques to help them adapt or function more independently in their environment.	
PF.1.7. Patients are taught that pain management is a part of treatment.[a]	
PF.1.8. Patients are informed about access to additional resources in the community.	
PF.1.9. Patients are informed about when and how to obtain any further treatment the patients may need.	
PF.1.10. The hospital makes clear to patients and families what their responsibilities are regarding the patients' ongoing health care needs and gives them the knowledge and skills they need to carry out their responsibilities.	

PF.1.11 With due regard for privacy, the hospital teaches and helps patients maintain good standards for personal hygiene and grooming, including bathing, brushing teeth, caring for hair and nails, and using the toilet.

Helpful chapters are the same as those mentioned for PF.1.3-PF.1.7.

PF.2. Patient education is interactive.

Although the entire book is based on interactive partnerships between patients and providers, several chapters emphasize interaction in particular. Chapter 1, "How Do I Know What Patients Want and Need?" and Chapter 3, "Do I Know Where to Go, and Will I Know When I Get There?" discuss mechanisms for gathering information from patients and providers. Chapter 4, "How Do I Get From a Needs Assessment to a Program?" defines an interactive planning process and teaching methods that are participative. Chapter 9, "The Special Problem of Compliance," describes an interactive process to help patients address compliance issues.

PF.3. When the hospital gives discharge instructions to the patient or family, it also provides these instructions to the organization or individual responsible for the patient's continuing care.

Chapter 7, "Selecting, Preparing, and Using Materials," and Chapter 6, "Working Cross-Culturally," provide guidance on the development of discharge materials. Chapter 9, "The Special Problem of Compliance," offers insight into how to help patients address compliance issues when they are at home.

PF.4. The hospital plans, supports, and coordinates activities and resources for patient and family education.

Chapters 1, 4, and 7 address critical issues in planning patient education activities—needs assessment, evaluation, and program implementation. Chapter 5, "How Do I Get People to Come?" focuses on marketing strategies to encourage referrals from health professionals and participation by patients and families.

continued

TABLE 10.1 Continued

JCAHO Education Standard	Helpful Chapters
PF.4.1. The hospital identifies and provides the educational resources required to achieve its educational objectives.	Chapters 4, 6, and 7 address the resources needed to achieve educational objectives.
PF.4.2. The patient and family educational process is collaborative and interdisciplinary, as appropriate to the plan of care.	Chapter 1, "How Do I Know What Patients Want and Need?" describes strategies for collecting information from all stakeholders—patients, families, and health professionals. Chapter 4, "How Do I Get From a Needs Assessment to a Program?" addresses the importance of collaboration in program development. Chapter 5, "How Do I Get People to Come?" encourages further linkages with other health professionals and community organizations.

SOURCE: The JCAHO standards are reprinted with permission from Joint Commission on Accreditation of Healthcare Organizations, *CAMH: Comprehensive Accreditation Manual for Hospitals*, copyright 1999 by the Joint Commission on Accreditation of Healthcare Organizations, Oakbrook Terrace, IL.

a. Standards related to pain assessment and management will not be scored for compliance in the year 2000, but rather at a later date still to be determined.

It should be noted that other sections of the accreditation manual include standards that are related to patient education. For example, the chapter "Assessment of Patients" includes a standard mandating a psychosocial assessment; a standard in the chapter titled "Continuum of Care" specifies that patients should receive information about their proposed care plans. Still other chapters add related topics. The chapter titled "Patient Rights and Organizational Ethics" addresses patients' rights, participation in care, and advance directives; "Management of the Environment for Care" deals with the maintenance of an environment that fosters positive self-image for the patient and a nonsmoking policy; "Management of Information" addresses the availability of systems and resources to support education services; and "Management of Human Resources" addresses the maintenance of staff competencies.

For the year 2000, standards related to a comprehensive approach to pain management have been integrated broadly into all accreditation programs, although they will not be scored for compliance until a future date. The broad scope of these standards suggests that all health-related organizations should gear up for a systemwide approach to pain. The Veterans Health Administration, for example, has recently launched a comprehensive national pain management strategy with the release of a "tool kit" for implementation of the administration's program titled *Pain Assessment, the 5th Vital Sign* (1999).

Further changes are expected in the format, if not the intent, of the education standards in future years as JCAHO introduces core and program-specific accreditation standards for all of its accreditation programs—hospitals, home care, ambulatory care, behavioral health, and long-term care. These will include (a) core standards for education planning that address the organization's planning and resource-procurement processes; (b) core standards for individual education, such as education about how to use medications safely and effectively; and (c) accreditation-program-specific individual education standards.

Most health care organizations are now well aware of the changes related to patient education standards. Thus you are likely to begin planning well in advance for JCAHO visits. This planning often includes the use of systemwide committees, mock surveys, staff training, and other strategies to prepare for the accreditation visit. Although chart documentation, patient assessment, and policy availability continue to be surveyed, you may also want to plan for some of the special patient education issues emphasized during recent visits. These have included the following:

- *Interdisciplinary versus multidisciplinary:* Surveyors continue to emphasize the interdisciplinary rather than the merely multidisciplinary. Are team members working together rather than by discipline to produce a treatment plan? Does your documentation of patient education reflect an integrated approach, or is it repetitious and reflective of the involvement of many separate disciplines? For example, are your courses a combination of integrated content and process, or are they lecture series with a different health professional talking about a different topic each week?

- *Continuity of care:* As your patients receive care in an increasingly diverse array of settings, what mechanisms do you have in place to ensure that the information provided in the home, the hospital, the clinic, and the long-term care setting is consistent? How does a clinician in your outpatient setting know what has been provided by the home care nurse, for example, or vice versa?

- *Quality improvement focus:* Surveyors want to know that you have assessed outcomes of care in order to address ongoing problems and assure that quality of care is maintained. JCAHO is currently pilot testing a standardized performance measure initiative that will eventually require organizations to collect specified process and outcome data. Some of the measures are very treatment oriented, whereas others, such as the provision of smoking cessation counseling to myocardial infarction patients, address educational needs.

- *Resources for special populations:* Surveyors are interested in seeing that providers have gone beyond assessing cultural or religious preferences and have resources to address identified needs. Do you have lists of interpreters available? Are there diabetic exchange lists for different groups of ethnic foods? Do you have available written materials, audio- and videotapes, and lists of Internet sites directed to the needs of local cultural and religious groups?

- *Alternative and complementary therapies:* Consumers have a growing interest in alternative therapies. In addition, there is a growing research base related to such therapies. Thus surveyors would like you to have appropriate teaching materials concerning alternative and complementary therapies available for patients. Patient learning centers and information kiosks are good sources, and some inpatient units have special carts stocked with distraction therapies for pain management; cancer treatment or ambulatory surgery centers may offer relaxation tapes to reduce chemotherapy side effects and preoperative anxiety.

- *Pain management:* These new standards are receiving substantial emphasis as surveyors encourage broad thinking about pain initiatives in health care organizations. How do you enable patients to talk about and assess their pain? Are clinicians prepared to answer patient concerns? What resources are available to help patients manage pain? How are families involved?

Finally, depending on the format of your accreditation site visit, you may want to take advantage of this opportunity to help the surveyors understand directly how patient education works. At some health care organizations, the patient education interview is experiential, with site visitors participating in a brief introduction and assessment in the patient learning center that model the intake process for a new patient. At other organizations where patients sit on patient education committees, these patients have participated in site visits, showcasing consumer involvement and community participation. At still other sites, the commitment to active patient education is visually apparent in the organization through the use of posters, bulletin boards, pamphlets, videos, special education carts, and logos.

Please note that this chapter was written in 2000, and that changes may have occurred since publication of this volume. For updated information on accreditation standards and related issues, check the JCAHO Web site at http://www.jcaho.org. The site not only provides information on forthcoming changes in standards and the accreditation process but makes phone numbers and e-mail addresses available to facilitate your obtaining answers to specific questions.

✪ BIBLIOGRAPHY

American Hospital Association. (1979). *Implementing patient education in the hospital.* Chicago: Author.

Deeds, S. G., Hebert, B. J., & Wolle, J. M. (Eds.). (1979). *A model for patient education programming* (Special project report). Washington, DC: American Public Health Association, Public Health Education Section.

Giloth, B. E. (Ed.). (1993). *Managing hospital-based patient education.* Chicago: American Hospital Association.

Joint Commission on Accreditation of Healthcare Organizations. (1999). *CAMH: Comprehensive accreditation manual for hospitals.* Oakbrook Terrace, IL: Author.

Veterans Health Administration, Acute Care Strategic Healthcare Group & Geriatric/Extended Care Strategic Healthcare Group. (1999). *Pain assessment, the 5th vital sign.* Washington, DC: Author.

Glossary

Acculturation The process by which one acquires the values, practices, and language of another culture.

Adherence *See* **Compliance.**

Assimilation The extreme form of acculturation, in which one loses one's cultural practices of origin and completely acquires and adopts a new culture.

Back-translation A method of translation that uses two independent translators. The first translator translates the material from the original language to the new language; the second translator takes the translated material and translates it back into the original language. The two original-language versions are then compared to judge the accuracy and appropriateness of the translation.

Balanced incomplete block design A technique for quantifying and prioritizing qualitative data.

Brainstorming A technique by which a group generates as many ideas as possible without placing comment or value on the ideas generated.

229

Comparison group Subjects chosen to be compared with the treatment subjects in a nonrandom manner.

Compliance (adherence) Following directions.

Cultural diversity The result of interactions between different cultures.

Cultural identity The culture or cultures with which one identifies at any specific time.

Culture A shared set of beliefs, assumptions, values, and practices.

Educational needs assessment Determination, in a planned manner, of the perceived needs of patients, their significant others, providers, or all of these concerning health.

Epi Info A user-friendly, inexpensive data management and statistical analysis software package.

Focus group A group interviewed to obtain information on specific ideas or concerns.

Formative evaluation *See* **Process evaluation.**

Hard-to-reach people People or patients health educators have problems reaching because of environmental, cultural, or other mediating factors.

Health behavior Any action one takes to maintain or improve health, to prevent disease, or to slow physical or emotional decline.

Health care utilization The frequency with which one uses health care providers or institutions—for example, nights in hospital, number of outpatient visits to a physician, or number of home care visits.

Health status One's current physical or emotional functioning. Usually measured in terms of pain, disability, depression, shortness of breath, fatigue, and so on; can also be measured by self-rated overall health.

Measurement instrument *See* **Scale.**

Model A plan or way of organizing things.

Objective data Data that are unbiased; often data that can be verified against another source.

Operational definition Definition of a term for any specific study or context. For example, see **Patient education** for the operational definition of this term as it is used in this book.

Outcome evaluation (also known as **summative evaluation**) An evaluation of how well the objectives of the program were met. Outcomes are usually measured in terms of health behaviors, health status, and/or health care utilization.

Patient A person who has a defined and present health problem.

Patient education A set of planned educational activities designed to improve patients' health behaviors and/or health status.

Process evaluation (also known as **formative evaluation**) An evaluation of what goes on during and sometimes before a health education intervention–for example, how many people came or whether the intervention was delivered as written.

Qualitative data Data that are usually in text form, usually descriptive.

Quantitative data Data that are usually in numeric form; data that can be manipulated statistically.

Questionnaire If the questionnaire is measuring only one construct–for example, pain–then it is the same as a scale or a measurement instrument. Sometimes a questionnaire is composed of many scales.

Randomized Assigned to one group or another (usually treatment and control) in no particular order and with no specific purpose.

Rationale A statement of reasons.

Readability Capability of being read and understood. Adults may be able to read well above their tested levels of reading comprehension if the information is important to them.

Rehearsal Practicing of what to say or how to act in a potentially problematic situation before it occurs.

Role playing Acting out a situation or interaction in a safe environment.

Salient beliefs The most important beliefs one holds about any given subject.

Scale (also known as **measurement instrument**) A collection of items or questions used to find out something specific that is not directly observable.

Self-management Being responsible for and making decisions about one's health. This includes monitoring one's health, making informed decisions about when to use health care providers, practicing appropriate health behaviors, using a problem-solving approach to make decisions, and using family, friends, and community resources as appropriate and necessary.

Self-monitoring Keeping track of one's symptoms or behaviors. The information from self-monitoring is often used to make decisions about medications or health behaviors.

Sensitivity The degree to which a scale or instrument responds to change. If it responds only to large changes, it is not very sensitive. If it responds to small changes, it is sensitive.

Subjective data Data coming from one's mind; these data often cannot be verified against an outside source.

Summative evaluation *See* **Outcome evaluation.**

Theory A system of ideas used to explain a particular phenomenon.

Validity Truthfulness or correctness of the measurement of what the evaluator wants to measure.

Index

About the Author

Kate Lorig, Dr.P.H., R.N., is Associate Professor (Research) at Stanford University School of Medicine and is also Director of the Stanford Patient Education Research Center. She has spent the past 22 years developing and evaluating community-based patient education programs for people with chronic diseases. She has also acted as a consultant for major health maintenance organizations, hospitals, and voluntary health agencies. Her programs have been adapted in several countries, including Canada, Australia, New Zealand, Great Britain, South Africa, Norway, and China.

About the Contributing Coauthors

Cecilia Doak, M.P.H., is, with Leonard Doak, a founder of Patient Learning Associates, Inc., and is one of the foremost experts in the United States on the preparation of health education materials.

Leonard Doak, B.S., P.E., is, with Cecilia Doak, a founder of Patient Learning Associates, Inc., and is one of the foremost experts in the United States on the preparation of health education materials.

Barbara E. Giloth, Dr.P.H., C.H.E.S., is currently Director of the Foundation and Community Benefit Progams, Advocate Charitable Foundation, Advocate Health Care. She has previously held positions as an independent health care consultant, as a director, health services research at HRET and as a program manager at the American Hospital Association.

Virginia M. González, M.P.H., is a Research Assistant at the Stanford Patient Education Research Center. She received her M.P.H. from the University of California at Berkeley.

Lynn Gordon is a writer, editor and translator. She specializes in health education and low-literacy materials.

Margo Harris is a school and community specialist with Harris Training & Consulting Services in Seattle. She works closely with school districts and community organizations to improve health instruction and patient education. To learn more about her, visit www.htcs.com/margo.htm

Thomas R. Prohaska, Ph.D., is Professor and Director of the Division of Community Health Sciences at the University of Illinois at Chicago (UIC) School of Public Health and Codirector of the University of Illinois Center for Research on Health and Aging. His research interests focus on gerontological public health including health behavior, illness behavior in older adults, and the psychosocial factors associated with self-care in older populations.